COMPLETE GUIDE TO TOTAL

HEALTH AND WELLNESS

What you need to know about

diet, exercise and stress management

Daniel A. Lonquist, DC, CCST, CCWP

Greg Haitz, DC, CCSP

DISCLAIMER

The information contained in this book is provided solely for educational purposes. It is not a substitute for medical advice. Always consult with your own healthcare provider regarding your medications, medical conditions and treatments.

ABOUT THE AUTHORS

Dr. Daniel Lonquist

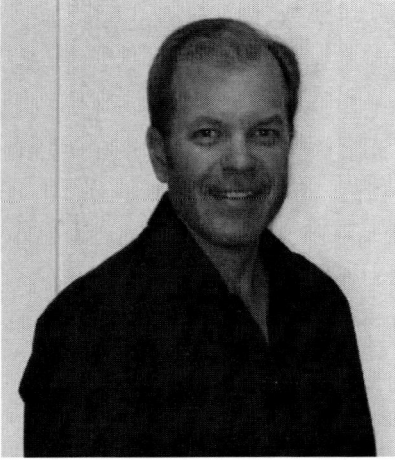

Dr. Daniel Lonquist has had a passion for fitness and health from a young age. This has been reflected in his personal lifestyle, graduate studies, and career choice. Prior to completing his doctor of Chiropractic degree at Western States Chiropractic College in Portland, Oregon, Dr. Lonquist attended the University of British Columbia, the University of Alberta and Simon Fraser University. He received a Bachelor of Science degree in Kinesiology, the study of human movement and performance. Before moving to Colorado in 1996, Dr. Lonquist practiced in Vancouver, British Columbia where he also served as a member of the Chiropractic College Licensing Board. Dr. Lonquist has continued his postgraduate studies in Colorado earning a specialty in the treatment of spinal trauma and certification as a wellness practitioner. Currently he is the only practitioner holding this honor in all of Western Colorado. When not working with patients to improve their health and wellness at his busy practice, he keeps physically active with a cross section of sports such as skiing, tennis, running, hiking and racquetball, in particular. He is also an avid reader and committed to staying informed on the latest research in health and wellness.

Dr. Greg Haitz

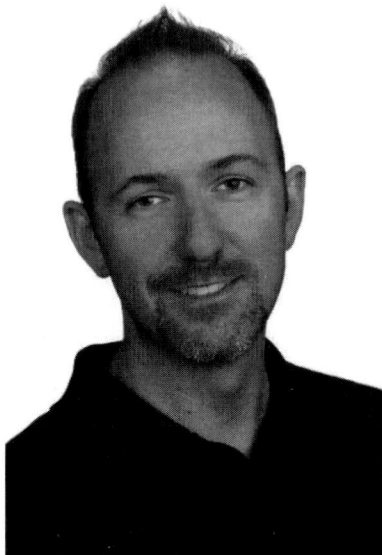

Dr. Greg Haitz first became interested in health and wellness at a young age. He would often find himself reading food labels and nutritional facts. As a teenager, he studied exercise, nutrition, and weight training. These early interests persisted as he pursued college studies in biology, psychology, and exercise at Mesa State College in Grand Junction, Colorado. Upon finishing his studies at Mesa State, Dr. Haitz was accepted into the prestigious Palmer College of Chiropractic in Iowa where he graduated with a Bachelor of Science degree and Doctor of Chiropractic degree in 2003. He also completed an internship in the Palmer College Sports Injury and Rehab Department. Dr. Haitz opened Rimrock Chiropractic, a creating wellness center in Grand Junction, Colorado to help his clients live a healthier lifestyle. By addressing the dimensions of physical, biochemical and psychological stress, he incorporates fitness and exercise, weight management and nutrition, stress management, and the mind/ body connection in helping his clients make healthier lifestyle choices. Dr. Haitz was nominated for the Colorado Rising Star Chiropractor of the Year in 2009 and has lectured extensively in his community on diet, nutrition, fitness and wellness.

Acknowledgement

Many people have helped with this book and I would like to thank all of them, however, there are a few I want to specifically mention. For the exercise portions of this book I want to thank Kiele Wilson and Stacy Antonnucci. Both of you were tremendous in helping to develop efficient exercise routines that can be done with limited equipment.

I would like to thank my aunt, Eija for helping to transcribe our first few online modules.

Most importantly I want to thank my mother, Raya for the countless hours transcribing the remaining online modules and contributing to our Wellness Solution books. I also want to thank her for constantly pushing me further and inspiring me to be the best I can be.

Daniel Lonquist

Table of Contents

Introduction

Hello and welcome to *The Complete Guide to Total Health and Wellness: What you need to know about diet, exercise and stress management*. This book is designed to help people know what they need to promote wellness and to improve their health and that of their family's over the course of their lives.

It can be confusing out there. Every day we hear something about health and wellness that either conflicts with what we thought we knew or is a new concept we were unaware of. This book will guide you through urban legends and misinformation being promoted today as health and wellness.

Treating disease once it shows up has not been an effective strategy in health care. Together, Dr. Lonquist and Dr. Haitz have a mission to take their experience and approach as field doctors, and bring it to everyone. Although they've discovered simple and attainable secrets to health and wellness, it has been impossible for them to reach everyone – until now. This guide covers the aspects of health and wellness that you need to know to strive for optimal health. Utilizing the included education and tools, it will be as if you have access to your own exercise and fitness professional, nutritionist, and stress management lifestyle coach – all wrapped up and delivered in an easy and convenient guide.

With the rise in obesity, lack of fitness and pervasive stress, we need to proactively address lifestyle issues and prevention.

Synopsis

This book is a compilation of the 12 books in our *Wellness Solution Series*. Each of the books in that series has become a chapter in this book. Here is a synopsis of each chapter.

- Chapter 1, *How to Achieve Optimal Health & Wellness*, establishes parameters for what health and wellness are as they relate to emotional, physical and biochemical goals.

- Chapter 2 is *Testing Your Health:* Are You Healthy? It shows you how to set some baseline scores towards your personal wellness objectives.
- Chapter 3, *Nutrition and Exercise Fundamentals,* focuses on nutrition and exercise basics.
- Chapter 4, *From Toxic to Clean and Lean, looks* at turning toxicities and deficiencies into purity and sufficiency.
- Chapter 5, *Demystifying Medications, Supplements and Common Diseases* addresses supplements and medication.
- Chapter 6, *The Hidden Truth about Diet and Nutrition* discusses what is meant by a good diet.
- Chapter 7, *Eat Clean and Regain Your Health* examines the importance of periodically cleansing your body of toxins.
- Chapter 8 explores *Eating Well: Aspects of Health and Wellness* and includes a recipe book.
- Chapter 9 focused on Exercise for Optimal Wellness.
- In Chapter 10, *Mind Body Healing: How to Create Optimal Health Using Your Thoughts,* we talk about the mind-body connection and how to manage our stress using various simple techniques.
- Chapter 11, *The Nervous System and Wellness: Understanding How They Relate Will Lead Towards Optimal Health*, we discuss in a simple and easy to understand way, how the nervous system works. Health issues are often connected to assaults on the nervous system. Our bodies interface with the world through our nervous system. We discuss how to determine if you have nerve interference and what you can do to remove it.
- Chapter 12, *The Power of Attraction: Simple Steps to Achieve Your Dreams, Wishes and Goals,* gives you techniques to discover your purpose so you will be able start attracting your dreams, wishes and goals through the power of attraction.

Chapter 1

How to Achieve Optimal Health and Wellness

What is Health?

If you were to ask a group of people what health is you'd probably get a lot of different answers. Some might say it's how they feel or that they don't have any diseases. The problem is, this doesn't really encapsulate what true health is.

Health is... "A condition of wholeness in which all the tissues, organs and systems of the body are functioning 100% of the time." – Webster's Dictionary

Health is more than just feeling well and more than the absence of disease. It is about function. For instance, a person can feel great but still have a problem. Of all heart attacks, 50% happen with no prior symptoms. Yet, heart disease is a condition that develops over years and years. Those people were not healthy even though they were feeling well. Conversely, a person can feel quite poorly and yet be healthy. When people catch a cold, for instance, they say that they're sick. However, feeling sick is a healthy expression of the body fighting off a cold virus.

So, how do you know if you're healthy and how do you know if you have wellness? In 1996, Lance Armstrong competed in triathlons, cycled, ate well and felt good. Then one day he had to pull out of a competition because he wasn't feeling right. After running a bunch of tests, the doctor announced he had testicular cancer that had metastasized to his brain and to his lungs. Here was an individual that, on the outside, looked healthy. On the inside, however, cancer was growing in his body. To rely on symptoms as an indication of health could lead to big trouble. Once the "check engine" light comes on in your car's dashboard, it indicates that something is already broken. If we are waiting for indicators to show up in our health, we're going to be pretty broken and require some major intervention. Unfortunately, that's what the approach

3

has been in US health care. That's not creating health, that's just treating disease.

What is Wellness?

Wellness is one of those buzz words right now. We hear a lot about wellness but it's hard to define. Is it drinking bottled water? Jogging? Taking vitamins? Is it all those together? While those things are beneficial, wellness encompasses more than that. The idea of wellness is the degree to which we experience health and vitality in any dimension of our lives.

This definition allows a person to always be working on wellness and working toward wellness. When we think about our lives, there are basically three dimensions in which we live.

1. The Physical Dimension: What we do with our bodies physically and how we relate to our environment using our five senses?

2. The Biochemical Dimension: What chemical interactions do we have, both inside and outside our body, i.e., the shampoo we put on our heads, the water we drink, and the quality of the air we breathe?

3. The Emotional Dimension: What is happening psychologically—how do we think about certain things and how we feel emotionally?

The degree to which an individual experiences health and vitality in any one dimension can vary. For example, it's possible to experience excellent physical health while experiencing poor emotional health. Likewise, a person might have the biochemical aspect of their life completely figured out – eating organic foods, drinking good water, living in a climate that doesn't have much pollution – but at the same time, may not be physically exercising like they should, have poor posture, etc. Viewing wellness in various dimensions, gives the opportunity to build wellness in parts of one's life while still working on others. Wellness is a continuum. We're either moving toward or away from it based on the decisions we make. When we wake up in the morning, we're making a daily decision, "Am I going to have a donut for breakfast or am I going to have a smoothie?" One is a disease decision and one is a wellness decision. "Am I going to sit in my office chair all day long with poor posture or am I going to sit up straight and get up every thirty minutes and walk around?" Again, one is a disease decision; one is a wellness decision. If we're ever going to reach a point of wellness, we're going to have to head toward wellness. If we're not, we'll be heading toward disease or sickness.

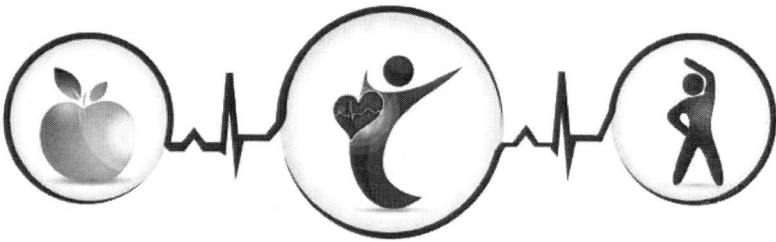

Three Dimensions of Wellness

Let's start with the physical dimension. In this dimension, we encounter positive stress and negative stress. Negative stress can range from simple traumas like stubbing our toe, to experiencing a major car accident, or to giving birth. Even the little tumbles that we take as children, however, tend to accumulate in our bodies. In fact, the typical adult will encounter approximately 240 physical traumas per year.

In addition, there are physical stresses we don't often think about – like repetitive strain injuries. Working in an environment using a mouse and keyboard all day when their position isn't ergonomically correct is a good example. Over time, this can create a physical stress that our bodies must to adapt to.

On the other hand, our bodies can experience positive physical stresses like exercise, stretching, and even fiber in our diet moving through our intestine. These are examples of good, positive, and necessary physical stresses that our bodies encounter and grow through.

Biochemical stress is a category many don't think about. It represents all the different chemicals and toxins we assimilate into our bodies as we interact with our environment. Air pollution is one example. If you live in Chicago, for instance, there's a high level of pollution. Studies show air pollution has a lot to do with incidences of MS and other neurological disorders. Pollution is a big deal. Our bodies must adapt to that biochemistry.

Although our bodies are always adapting to the environment, it's when they have trouble adapting to additional stress that we start to encounter problems.

Fast food, too much coffee, and energy drinks can alter the biochemistry of our bodies and force them to adapt. If we put too much sugar into our bodies at one time, it spikes our blood sugar requiring the pancreas to release insulin in order to drop the blood sugar level and push the sugar into our cells. Our cells then, store it as fat for fuel.

Toxins like radon gas or even those found in hairspray can also put stress on the body. In some areas of the country, there's radon gas that comes up from the ground into the home. This has been quoted as the second leading cause of lung cancer today. Yet, as bad as radon is, we put petroleum bi-products in our make-up, hairspray, and fingernail polish. All these chemicals can become quite toxic and require our bodies to break them down through the liver. Even pharmaceutical medications and prescription drugs have harsh chemicals in them that our bodies must adapt to and break down.

Emotional stress can often be the most deleterious when it comes to our health. Even though we don't think about our emotional health as having anything to do with our bodies, it's really that mind/body connection where our bodies are forced to deal with emotional stress. These can result from a sudden emotional incident or from something that happens gradually over time.

Losing a loved one suddenly, whether through natural causes or something like a car accident, would produce an abrupt emotional stress. Although the incident was sudden, the emotional stress could be present in the body for years to come.

Other long-term emotional stresses could be experiencing abuse as a child, dealing with an overbearing parent, verbal abuse in the home, or even a protracted divorce. Anyone who's been through a divorce understands what it's like to go through months of emotional stress. This kind of strain can break down the body – in both children and adults. Whether it's a difficulty with a spouse, a child, or a crazy teenager, it's these constant emotional stresses that can put us in a state of turmoil. Even if our health in the physical and biochemical dimensions is functioning well, in the emotional arena we can simply be a wreck. Therefore, in terms of total wellness, we can be experiencing some level of wellness in one or more dimensions while experiencing serious deficiencies in the others.

Although we encounter many negative biochemical stresses in our environment, there are also positive ones. Good, clean drinking water, good fiber in our diet, phytochemicals, and enzymes in our foods are good biochemical stressors that cause growth and change in our bodies.

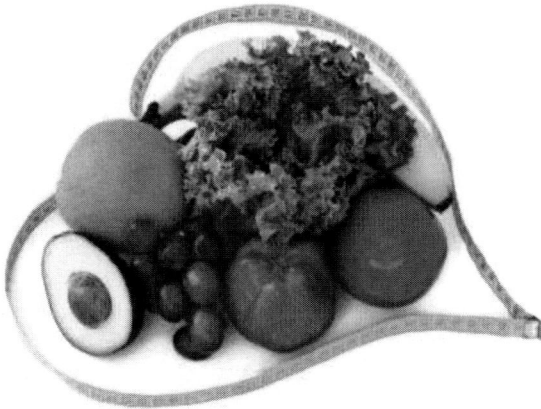

Our Current State of Health

In the United States, we currently spend more money on health care than any country in the world. We also take 75% of the world's medications, get the most surgeries, and have the most state-of-the-art equipment. It would seem that this would translate to a healthy population. However, treating disease and creating health and wellness are two different roads. Although we spend the most money on health care, our ranking is 37th in the world for healthcare systems, according to World Health Organization, and we're 13th in the world for preventable diseases. In other words, we're dying from diseases that could be prevented. This means we're good at treating disease but we are not good at creating health and wellness. In addition, we're 38th in the world for life expectancy at birth. With the type of technology we have, that's unacceptable. We're literally killing ourselves.

If you get in a car accident and your leg is bleeding, you probably don't need to eat an apple, drink distilled water, or go for a run. That's not going to fix the problem. You need to go to an emergency room and let the qualified health professionals attend to your injuries. At the same time, you don't go to an emergency room to create health and wellness. The system is not designed for that. Furthermore, when we consider health insurance, it functions more as disease insurance. If disease shows up in our bodies, insurance is there to help. However, it's not designed to help us produce health and wellness in our lives. That's a much more personal decision and a personal responsibility.

Our health care system is misdefined. It should be considered more of a sick-care system.

The Leading Causes of Death

Of the four leading causes of death, the top three are lifestyle-based diseases. There is a notion that it's all in a person's genes. If a person's mom had heart disease, for example, and her mom had heart disease, and that person's dad died of a heart attack, it means he/she is destined to have heart disease. If that's true, why try? The problem with that thinking is that yes, it's true that we can carry certain tendencies in our genetics. If our parents had bad knees, the likelihood of us having bad knees is fairly high – unless we make some specific lifestyle choices to ensure that does not happen. There's a body of medical research that shows our lifestyle can either turn on or turn off certain genes. A good lifestyle has been shown to turn off cancer causing genes. This is very exciting. These types of diseases are all preventable. When we look at heart disease, there are over 600,000 deaths per year – due primarily to how we're living our lives. We didn't see these statistics a hundred years ago. Though our genes haven't changed during that period of time, our lifestyle certainly has.

As we look at the three leading causes of death, we realize they're all lifestyle-based. Heart disease, cancer, and stroke are all based on our body's inability to adapt to certain stresses caused by poor diet, insufficient exercise, and not managing our emotional stress appropriately.

The fourth leading cause of death is a bit surprising. It's medications. This is not a case of some child taking the parents' prescription pills from the medicine cabinet. It's a case of an adverse reaction to a properly prescribed medication. This is an individual with a medical condition who goes to a doctor, gets a prescription, takes it as prescribed, and dies. Most of the statistics we're seeing now indicate medications are easily number four on the list – maybe higher. That's a scary realization because those are deaths due to our current health care system.

Interestingly, if you look on the Center for Disease Control (CDC) website for statistics relating the leading causes of death to medications, it isn't even listed there. However, it's unlikely that they're purposely trying to hide information. More likely, they are listing what a person actually dies from. If one has an adverse drug reaction it might cause respiratory failure so that's what's listed.

This doesn't mean that medications aren't valuable or necessary in certain circumstances. However, it would be far more beneficial if we could prevent the need for those medications in the first place.

When we look at the first three causes of death, we can be assured that all those conditions will be medicated in a manner similar to the way other chronic diseases are treated. Most pharmaceutical companies spend the bulk of their research money on chronic diseases because those are the ones that aren't easily cured and are going to be treated for the length of a person's life. For instance, acid reflux, gout, and glaucoma are types of diseases requiring medication for a person's entire life. As a result, the risk of having an adverse drug reaction increases. Based on that risk, we rank medications as the number four leading cause of death.

People don't receive accurate statistics of what is causing death. It's dangerously misleading. The real issue is that people are dying from medications and it's not being presented to the public appropriately.

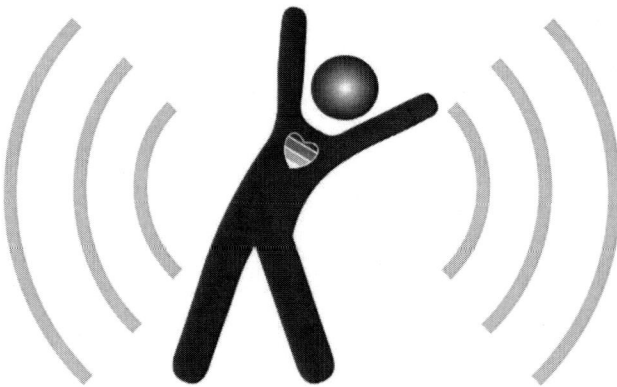

Type 2 Diabetes

The incidences of type 2 diabetes are increasing every year. Although there may be a predisposition for people acquiring it, most agree that it is a lifestyle-based disease.

It's likely to be the next big epidemic. The most recent statistics from the CDC show that about 11% of twenty-year old individuals have type 2 diabetes. That's alarming and outrageous since it's a 100% preventable disease. It's lifestyle that determines how one's body is going to express itself and whether that disease will manifest itself or not. What it comes down to is diet. A steady intake of refined carbohydrates and simple sugars, day in and day out, produces a dangerous cycle.

Type 2 diabetes is a silent killer. It slowly develops, doing damage over years and years. For some individuals, the first symptom might be vision problems or numbness and tingling in their arms or feet. These can be signs of nerve damage from diabetes. Years ago, if a person went outside and urinated and saw a bunch of ants collect around the urine, it meant they had "sugar diabetes." The problem is, type 2 diabetes is a lifestyle disease that develops slowly over time.

Testing for disease, however, isn't the same as preventing disease. Again, those are two different roads. Creating a healthy lifestyle is a lot different than waiting for disease to show up and then trying to treat it. If you simply wait until Type 2 diabetes shows up, it can be difficult to reverse. Although it can be done, the process can be arduous due to the years it's taken to develop.

When blood sugar continually elevates and crashes back down, our cells become resistant to insulin. When this happens, the sugars in our blood system aren't cleared properly. Over time, that sugar in our blood can begin to damage cells – especially nerve cells.

Other Chronic Diseases

Among Americans, seven out of ten deaths are due to these chronic diseases. That's a surprising statistic that includes all deaths such as whether it's someone falling off their house and breaking their neck, someone getting into a car accident, or someone being murdered. The majority of deaths are due to chronic diseases.

Because of that, they play a major role in the US health crisis. Yet, these are preventable health problems. When seven out of ten deaths are preventable, that is catastrophic.

Statistics also indicate that one in every three adults is obese. That's not just being a little overweight. Once a person is ranked as obese the risk of heart disease, cancer, and stroke are magnified even more. Obesity is a type of chronic disease. In addition, one of every five youth between the ages of six and nineteen is considered obese. Listen to the news on any given night, it seems, and the media will be talking about how medical doctors are recommending that even children take cholesterol medication. Again, these are lifestyle diseases. This is a result of how these kids eat. A look at statistics from early 1980's indicates this wasn't always the case. However, as of the year 2000, 35% of the population was considered obese.

Not only do heart disease, stroke, cancer, and diabetes claim the majority of deaths, they are very costly because they can be drawn out over many years.

You may be surprised how simple it is to follow the suggestions in this guide. A few incremental steps on a regular day to day basis will go a long way in helping you reach your health and wellness goals.

We Are Living Longer, But...

In light of the fact that Americans are living longer, what kind of quality of life would you want if you knew you would live to be one hundred or more. Obviously, if a person is one hundred years old and has twenty chronic diseases, that would be a poor quality of life.

It's more than just living longer. It's about preventing chronic diseases along the way. Do you want to be active right up until the day you die or do you want to have your life prolonged without any quality?

Think of your oldest living relative – maybe your grandmother. Let's say she lived to be ninety-nine or one hundred years old. You're now sixty. Subtract your years from hers and that will indicate you have forty years remaining. If you have another forty years of chronic migraines, acid reflux, arthritis in your knees, insomnia, and sinus problems, it would make sense to start making some drastic changes. Maybe you're twenty or thirty years old without any diseases or symptoms yet. You potentially have another eighty years ahead of you. Again, the quality of those years is determined by how you live your life on a daily basis.

If we knew we were going to live to be one hundred years old, that should motivate us to make different lifestyle decisions so that we have quality in those years and not just quantity.

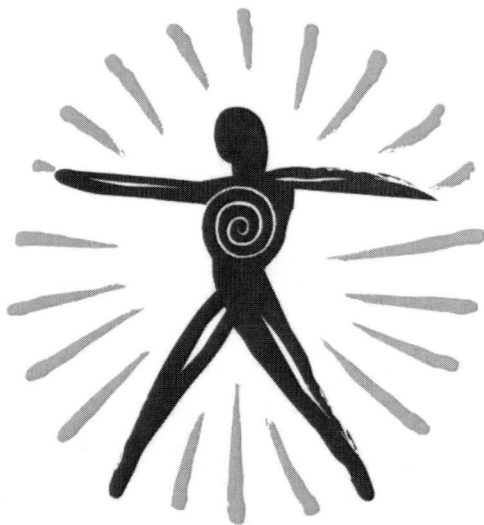

Let's go over everything we've discussed so far. We've related that health is not how we feel but about functioning. A person can feel fine and have disease or can feel terrible and still be fairly healthy. The closer a person gets to functioning at 100%, the healthier he/she is going to be. Likewise, wellness is measured by how we express our health and vitality in the physical, emotional, and biochemical dimensions. We know that putting more drugs and more surgery into our bodies isn't going to make us healthier. It's how we live that makes us healthier.

Lifestyle Crisis

In realty, we don't have a health care crisis, we have a lifestyle crisis. How we live right now is a lot different than how we lived a hundred years ago. It's not that medicine has failed us. It's that our lifestyle has shifted dramatically in the last fifty years and has created the health care crisis we see today. This means people need to make changes on an individual and personal basis.

The Honest Truth

The health care system isn't designed for health and isn't set up to be a health coach. Doctors can't administer health and wellness. Instead, we need to take very specific action steps. That's where The Wellness Connection comes in. It's no one else's responsibility to make us healthy. Health and wellness is a conscious effort that needs to be practiced on a daily basis throughout the day. Either we're moving toward wellness or moving toward disease. It needs to be a habit. You don't perform a lifestyle change once in a while. You don't just go to the gym once or twice a month and expect to be in peak physical condition. It needs to be part of your daily life. New Year's resolutions are not enough. They may be a way to kick-start habits again but New Year's resolutions never create health and wellness. It's what you do every single day that makes the difference.

What would you be willing to give to have more emotional freedom, happiness, energy, vitality, better sleep, and better digestion? By implementing very simple changes on a daily basis, it's possible to create a huge shift in how you function and feel. That's one reason we made this a year-long program. Any habit takes time to develop. Because wellness is a continuum, we need to constantly improve and implement new practices and disciplines.

30-Day Action Plan

In each section of this chapter will have different homework, different assignments, and different tools. In this particular part, we've discussed what health and wellness is and what it's not. Now we want to create a few action steps that can be done on a daily basis in the emotional, physical, and biochemical dimensions.

First, click on http://TheWellnessSolution.co/mod-1-downloads and print the PDF or make your own based on the following illustration.

30-Day Goal Sheet

Emotional Goal
Visualize the change you want to see 5-15 minutes per day, i.e. visualize your self doing activities at your ideal weight.

Physical Goal
Commit to an activity each day, i.e. take a walk around the block.

Biochemical Goal
Identify several chemical stressors in your life. Eliminate and replace one source per week, i.e. replace soda with water or green tea.

Put it somewhere you will see it every day. Next, write down what your goals are. On the emotional dimension, keep it fairly brief. Write down something you want to see change in your life.

Maybe you're seeking to have a better relationship with your spouse, child, or sibling. It may be a different interaction you'd like to see take place with your boss at work or maybe a role you would like to see yourself step into. It may be that you would like to start public speaking or take on a role in your church.

Whatever, the goal, you're going to visualize it every day – maybe first thing in the morning when you get up. Close your eyes and focus your mind's eye on doing that activity. Spend five, ten, or fifteen minutes visualizing those changes every day for thirty days. Let's say you want to visualize yourself at the weight you want to be. This would include visualizing how you're going to act when you're at that weight, the activities you'll be involved in, and the things you want to see. Simply visualize being whatever it is that you want to be. If you want to see yourself being physically fit, visualizing that will create changes in your habits and in your lifestyle.

Don't feel that this has to be perfect right now, it's simply a place to start. Obviously, a year from now we would hope that you'd still be doing your daily visualizations. What you visualize then will likely be different from what you're visualizing now. That's okay, this is just a place to start. What you visualize can even change daily.

What you visualize in your mind, your subconscious will start to believe and manifest in your life.

On the physical dimension, keep your activity simple as well. Commit to an activity every single day for the next thirty days. Maybe when you get home from work, you walk a half-mile around the block. If you're fairly active, it may be that you go to the gym three days a week. Maybe you do something like going to the gym five days a week and on the other couple of days, you go out for a two-mile walk. Maybe you take the stairs at work.

The important thing is that every single day you've got some sort of physical activity that you're doing. It's a matter of heading in the right direction. If you can't walk around the block it could be that you walk down the stairs. Whatever is an increase for you, just head in that direction for increasing your health and wellness.

If tomorrow you have better insight of where you want to be, it can be changed. It doesn't have to be a static thing.

On the biochemical aspect, identify some chemical stressors in your life and commit to eliminating those. Also, commit to replacing them with new sources. Maybe this week you just decide that you're not going to drink that soda and instead, you're going to replace it with something healthy like bottled water or green tea. Next week you may pick something else. You will want to keep that commitment throughout the rest of the month. That means that for the entire month, you're not going to drink soda. The following week you can decide to take on another biochemical stress. Maybe it's that morning donut that you're going to replace with a fruit smoothie.

Again, you'll make that change throughout the week and continue through the rest of the month. For the third week, do the same thing. Maybe you decide you want to replace your chemical dish soap with something that doesn't have all the harmful chemicals in it. Again, it's a process. It's a habit to continually think about and develop.

We're going to go into much more detail in future chapters regarding what these chemical stressors are and items you can replace them with. However, it's likely everyone can come up with four different stressors over the next month that they know would be much healthier if replaced with something else.

If you make a poor lifestyle choice every once in a while it's not going to kill you. If you do it every single day all throughout your day, that's a problem.

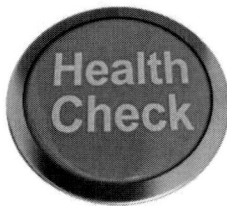

Now that we know what health and wellness are, we need to use some tools to establish a baseline. Then we can create a health and wellness road map to know where we want to go and how to get there.

It's very important to measure our objectives so we know if we're heading in the right direction.

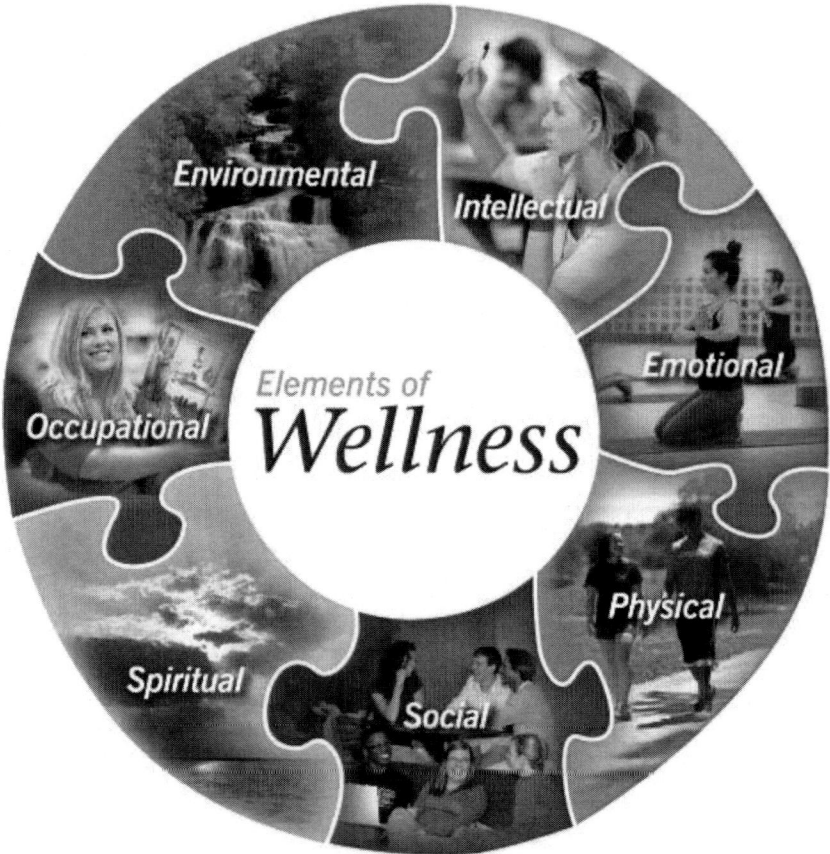

Elements of *Wellness*

Environmental

Intellectual

Emotional

Occupational

Physical

Spiritual

Social

Chapter 2
Testing Your Health: Are You Healthy?

So how do you determine whether you are healthy? To determine whether or not you are healthy, you first need to understand what is meant by *being healthy*. In a previous chapter, *How to Achieve Optimal Health & Wellness,* we established parameters for what health and wellness are. If you haven't already read the first chapter, it is recommended that you do so before proceeding to this second chapter of the Wellness Solution series.

Lifestyle, Genetics and Disease

In this chapter, we will provide you with some specific tests, online resources and questionnaires to assist you to assess your overall health and wellness. However, before we look at the specific tests, it's helpful to provide a brief discussion about lifestyle, epigenetics and disease.

The word 'epigenetics' is probably new for some people but it's becoming increasingly more mainstream. We are seeing it in a lot of medical literature so it will be helpful to provide a general overview of what it is to assist you to better understand the purpose of the selected tests and your test results.

Epigenetics looks at how our lifestyle affects our genes and the role of genetics in disease and health expression. The study of epigenetics is complex; therefore, it is not our intent to delve in depth into this area, but to simply point out that one's lifestyle and the environment one lives in plays a big role as to how our genes are expressed, and consequently you do have a choice as to whether you want to be healthy or not. Just because your parents or grandparents had a certain disease does not in any way mean that you will develop a similar illness. Your environment and how you take care of yourself can either increase or decrease your health and furthermore, it can influence the expression of your genes.

19

One good analogy is to compare genes to a blueprint similar to the blueprint of your house. If you have that blueprint stored somewhere, but you are not doing anything with it your house isn't going to be built. The environment has to take those instructions and do something with it. So, it's the same thing with our genes – it's our environment that influences that blueprint. That's the role of epigenetics in a nutshell - it's how that blueprint is expressed and what is done with it.

What about someone who has a family history of breast or prostate cancer? Suppose they have had genetic testing and they have been informed that they have the "breast or prostate cancer gene." What does someone like that need to do? If you implement some of the recommended strategies, will that make a difference? Will our diets, lifestyles or mind-sets make a difference as to whether the cancer gene will be expressed? What we mean by the term *expressed* is that our genes are either turned on or turned off like a blueprint. It's how our body's utilization of that certain genetic material will determine whether the gene ends up expressing a negative trait.

Dr. Bruce Harold Lipton, a developmental biologist has conducted a number of studies on this topic. He notes that if you take two identical cells and put them into two different petri dishes with a different environment, they could grow into two completely different things even though they have the same genes. So, in a different environment they're expressing something completely different.

It's worth noting that our genetics haven't changed much during the past forty thousand years, yet health issues such as heart disease have skyrocketed in the last hundred years. So, if our genes have remained virtually unchanged, what is causing this rapid acceleration? Is there a relationship between disease and lifestyle? We suggest that the answer to that is an unequivocal *yes!*

Research examining the remains of our hunter-gatherer ancestors suggests that they did not have osteoporosis or degenerative arthritis in their joints. Could it be that these diseases are a phenomenon that, in all likelihood, have taken place during the last hundred to hundred and fifty years or so?

Our genes were designed for a certain type of lifestyle? Perhaps it has taken these thousands of years for our genetics to be hardwired and adapted to that particular way of life. So, if our lifestyle has dramatically changed within a mere hundred-year window, that's a drop in the bucket compared to forty thousand years or so worth of genetic design. Consequently, it is understandable why our bodies cannot adequately adapt to our current lifestyle since our way of life is so extremely different from our original genetic blueprint. It's difficult for our bodies to adapt so quickly to an environment that has so significantly changed in such a short amount of time. In view of this reality, we need to focus on how we can change our lifestyle in our current circumstances to best sync with what our bodies were designed to do within our current environment.

Research examining the remains of our hunter-gatherer ancestors suggests that they did not have osteoporosis or degenerative arthritis in their joints.

Waist/Hip Ratio

The Waist to Hip Ratio test is also known as a *biometric test*. The nice thing about this test is that it's super simple to do in the comfort of your own home. Basically, all that is needed is a flexible tape measure, the kind you would buy in a fabric store. To test your waist to hip ratio simply find the widest circumference of the hips which is usually around the buttocks and take that measurement. Then take the smallest circumference around the waist which is usually around the belly button, maybe a lit bit above or a little bit below. It needs to be your natural waistline and not necessarily where you are wearing your jeans. Divide the waist number by the hip number. Research does suggest that people with more weight around the waist compared to the hips face increased health risks.

Waist/Hip Ratio

Hip measurement: widest part of the hips _____

Waist measurement: narrowest part of the waist, usually belly button or just below_____

Waist/Hip ratio _____
(Divide waist measurement by hip measurement.)

Waist/Hip Ratio (scores)

To find your waist/hip ratio score simply take your waist measurement divided by your hip measurement.

	Excellent	Good	Average	High	Extreme
Male	< 0.85	0.85 - 0.90	0.90 - 0.95	0.95 - 1.00	> 1.00
Female	< 0.75	0.75 - 0.80	0.80 - 0.85	0.85 - 0.90	> 0.90

(Example: male, waist 35 / hips 39 = .89 Good Healthy Range)

When you look at the difference between the male and female you're going to see a little bit of variation. It can range anywhere from excellent to good, average, high or extreme. In the example above, the 37-year-old male has a waist circumference of 35 and hip circumference of 39, so his waist ratio of .89 is considered a good healthy range according to the chart.

Although this is fairly basic, it's a baseline for you to start with. As you start progressing towards your health and wellness goals, you should begin to see a shift in your hip and waist ratios for the better.

Metabolic Typing

Another great test is called "Metabolic Typing," which is simply a test which looks at what types of foods that you eat will lead to optimal function of your body. For example, from what proportion of carbohydrates, fats and protein would your body benefit the most?

First, it's worth mentioning that there are good foods and bad foods. So, if you find out you are a "carbohydrate" metabolic type it doesn't mean that you can go out and eat a lot of bad carbs like candy, chocolate and things like that, however, there is a lot of research out there showing that some people, maybe through their genetics or for whatever reason function better with more of certain types of foods. This is a good tool to narrow down what type of foods might be better for your body type.

How you test should explain many things about your body type and food choices. Perhaps one of the best things about this test is that it may encourage you to pay more attention to what happens to your body when you eat certain foods, such as why you get fatigued an hour or two after eating. Of course, the point is not to get you caught up in your metabolic type as the be-all for health, but simply to see it as another useful tool to consider. This test should encourage you to start thinking more about what you eat which will undoubtedly move you closer towards the goal of reaching an elevated level of health and wellness.

Metabolic Typing

Adapted from The Metabolic Typing Diet (Wolcott and Fahey 2000, 135) and fatbellysolution.com

In the following 25 statements, circle the answer that best describes you. Answer according to how you feel, not how you think you should feel. If you don't have a good feel for how your body reacts to foods, pay attention for the next couple of days. Maybe even consider keeping a food diary to track how you feel after eating certain foods. To ensure a valid result, be honest and do not skip any questions!

1. When I am experiencing anxiety, anger, or irritability, eating . . .
A. Heavy fatty foods such as meat or nuts make me feel better.
B. Fruit, vegetables, or fruit juice makes me feel better.

2. I feel best when I eat the following for breakfast:
A. Sausage, eggs, bacon.
B. Cereal, fruit, oatmeal, and/or toast.

3. If I attended a buffet and could eat whatever I wanted (all health rules aside), I would choose
A. Steak, pork chops, ribs, gravy, and salad with creamy dressing.
B. Chicken, turkey, fish, vegetables, and a dessert.

4. I feel best when the temperature is
A. Cool or cold; I don't like hot weather.
B. Warm or hot; I don't like cold weather.

Metabolic Typing (continued)

5. Coffee makes me feel

A. Jittery, jumpy, nervous, hyper, shaky, or hungry.

B. Okay, as long as I don't drink too much.

6. In the morning, I am

A. Hungry and ready to eat breakfast.

B. Not hungry and don't feel like eating.

7. At midday, I am

A. Hungry and ready to eat lunch.

B. Not noticeably hungry and have to be reminded to eat.

8. In the evening, I am

A. Hungry and ready to eat dinner.

B. Not noticeably hungry and have to be reminded to eat.

9. I concentrate best if I have eaten a meal that includes

A. Meat and fatty foods.

B. Fruits, vegetables, and grains.

10. When I have cravings, I tend to want

A. Salty and fatty snacks (peanuts, cheese, or potato chips).

B. Baked goods or other carbs (bread, cereal, or crackers).

11. When I eat sugar or a sugary snack,

A. I feel a rush of energy, then am likely to crash and feel fatigued.

B. My energy levels are restored.

Metabolic Typing (continued)

12. If dessert is served,
A. I can take it or leave it; I would rather have cheese, chips, or popcorn.
B. I definitely will indulge; I like to have something sweet after a meal.

13. If I have a dessert, I most often choose
A. Cheesecake or creamy French pastries.
B. Cakes, cookies, or candies.

14. For dinner, I feel best (satiated) after eating
A. Steak and vegetables.
B. Skinless chicken breast, rice, and a salad.

15. I sleep best if my dinner is
A. Heavy and includes more proteins.
B. Light and includes more carbohydrates.

16. I wake up feeling well rested if
A. I don't eat sweets in the evening.
B. I eat sweets in the evening.

17. I feel best during the day if I eat
A. Small meals frequently, or three meals a day plus some snacks.
B. Two to three meals a day and no snacks; I can last pretty long without eating.

18. I describe myself as someone who
A. Loves to eat; food is a central part of my life.
B. Is not very concerned with food; I may forget to eat at times.

Metabolic Typing (continued)

19. If I skip a meal, I feel
A. Irritable, jittery, weak, tired, or depressed.
B. Okay; it doesn't really bother me.

20. If I had fruit and low-fat cottage cheese for lunch, I would feel
A. Hungry, irritable, and sleepy soon after.
B. Satisfied and probably could go until dinner after that.

21. During the day, I feel hungry
A. Often and need to eat several times a day.
B. Rarely and have a weak appetite.

22. I would describe myself as someone who is more
A. Extroverted—I am a very social person.
B. Introverted—I usually keep to myself.

23. When a food or meal is very salty,
A. I love it!
B. I don't enjoy it.

24. If I get hungry midafternoon, I feel best (more energized) after eating
A. Cheese and nuts.
B. Something sweet.

25. After exercising, I feel best if I eat
A. a protein shake or food that contains protein.
B. a high-sugar drink or food, such as a Gatorade or a banana.

Metabolic Typing (Scoring)

First, count how many times you circled A and B:

Total number of A answers = _____

Total number of B answers = _____

Next, referring to these scores, select your metabolism type classification according to the following criteria:

If your A score is 5 or more points higher than your B score (e.g., A = 15, B = 10), then you are a **Protein Type**.

If your B score is 5 or more points higher than your A score (e.g., A = 10, B = 15), then you are a **Carb Type**.

If your A and B scores are within 3 points of each other (e.g., A = 14, B = 11), then you are a **Mixed Type**.

Once you have gone through the **Metabolic Typing** questionnaire and tallied your scores, you are ready to select your metabolic type classification. The metabolic type test score is basically breaking down your results into three types, protein type, carb type or mixed type.

When we did ours, we both scored as mixed types, which didn't surprise us, but for many of you this might be a really good *uh huh* moment. If your 'A' score is five or more points higher than your 'B' score then you are a **Protein Type**. Also, if your 'B' score is five or more points higher than your 'A' score you're going to be more of a **Carb Type**. And then if your 'A' and 'B' scores are within three points of each other then you're basically a **Mixed Type**. This is simply a way to look at what you should be eating based on the information from a book by William (Bill) Wolcott called the

Metabolic Typing Diet. If people are interested in reading more about metabolic types, his book provides a useful reference.

Direct Labs: Comprehensive Wellness Profile

Some of you who may want more complete information about your overall health. For this you can conduct a comprehensive wellness profile that looks at areas such as cholesterol levels, blood count, white blood cells, red blood cells, thyroid and blood sugar levels. One option to consider is the nationwide company *Direct Labs* (http://www.Directlabs.com) that offers comprehensive wellness testing at reasonable prices. This particular lab offers the comprehensive wellness profile which includes fifty different tests that look at a broad range of overall health factors. Currently, only $97 - Over $450 savings off retail

The Direct Labs Wellness Panel includes Lipids Panel, Complete Blood Count, Thyroid Panel, Liver Panel, Kidney Panel, Minerals & Bones, Fluid & Electrolytes and Blood Sugar. The link to the Direct Labs Wellness Panel is http://www.directlabs.com/

You can retrieve the results online and there are some areas on the site where you can go and get interpretations as to what those results mean. Recently the FDA made a ruling that consumers can order their own blood work without having to go through a doctor and the results are confidential. These interpretations will be fairly generic but they will show if you are out of the normal ranges for these different panels such as cholesterol levels what that means.

Obviously, if you get your results back with some numbers that are elevated outside of the normal range or below the normal range, you should contact your family physician and have them review your results with you. But again, the benefit here is for someone who may not have insurance or a primary care doctor or who just wants to get a general overview of how their health looks from the lab blood analysis.

It's worth noting too that we are in no way associated with this lab. We simply found this lab a reasonably priced way to get a comprehensive blood profile done.

If there are some scores that are a little bit out of the normal range, by using lifestyle modification which is the focus of the Wellness Solution online program www.thewellnesssolution.co and this book, those levels should start coming back into the normal rage naturally. However, we do want to emphasize that if there are significant things out of the normal range you should be discussing this with your health care provider to determine if there are things that need to be done other than what we're recommending for general health and wellness.

Each day, you're either moving towards or away from wellness.

Daily Thought Exercise

What is your primary wellness goal? This daily thought exercise asks you to first clarify what you want and why you want it and then on a daily basis spend a few minutes in a focused and relaxed position thinking about having achieved your goal. You need to create a *burning desire* for what it is you want to achieve and not just, 'oh, it would be nice if I were healthier so I'm going to do this program.'

The idea behind the *Daily Thought Exercise* is simply to engage your conscious mind into focusing on a goal that you want to achieve. In order to attain your goal, you need to not only be clear as to what you want to achieve, but also believe that you will be able to achieve it. Are you wanting to be able to get into better shape so you can look and feel better? Do you simply want to have more energy to play with your kids? Or, are you just simply sick and tired of feeling sick and tired and are now finally determined to feel energetic and healthy?

Daily Thought Exercise

In order to be successful in anything, you need to know what you want. The following exercise will get you started.

1. Define specifically what you want. What is your dream? What is your goal? What is your desire? You can define it specifically or generally, e.g., I want a black Mercedes SL, with black leather interior. This would be specific. You could also just say I want a really nice car. This would be general. A third option would just be I want to feel really good every day when I leave my house. What makes you feel good is the best gauge for this exercise. It's about choosing a goal or thing that gives you the best feeling. Many times being general or just thinking about something that makes you "feel good" is the best way since there are often things that you would want more, you just haven't thought about them.

2. You must have a burning desire for it. It is not enough to just say want something. If you don't have a burning desire that makes you think about it all the time and with great intensity, it will often not come true.

3. You need to be thinking about it as often as possible for as long as possible and feel good about it and believe in it. If you don't believe it will happen, it won't! If you have trouble believing in something set smaller goals until you really believe you can achieve it. Don't worry about when it is going to happen.

4. You must believe in it and have no doubt. A good test to whether you believe it is that it should make you feel good when you think about it. If it doesn't, then you don't believe it will happen.

As a starting point to help you to define your goal, ask yourself what you want to achieve and why you want to achieve it. Creating a *burning desire* and spending a few minutes every day focusing on your goal is very important. You have to think about why you want something and to think about it on a daily basis.

This daily thought exercise could be done first thing in the morning by taking a few minutes to think about what you want. You could record your goal on a small piece of paper and laminate it, put it in your pocket, tape it in your shower, carry it around with you, put it in your car or anywhere to help you to think about it as many times as you can throughout the day and to get yourself motivated when you're thinking about it.

Of course, it is important to think about feeling good while you're thinking about your goal. This will help you to create a "yes I can achieve this" mind set. For instance, if your goal is to lose thirty pounds and get into shape, it's one thing to say, "I want to lose thirty pounds and get in shape", but it's a whole other thing to see in your mind's eye what you might look like and what you might feel like when you've lost that thirty pounds. Thinking about that is going to bring a smile to your face. When that happens, that burning desire, that believability is coming into play and that's an important part of the process.

Feeling good, as we mentioned is a good indicator in knowing whether you have a burning desire and whether you believe it's going to happen. If you believe what you want is going to happen, you're going to feel good when you are thinking about it. If for some reason you feel bad when you're thinking about it, deep down what that usually means is you don't believe it's going to happen so you get discouraged. If that's the case, you might have to modify your goal to make it a shorter goal or something that's more achievable for you. On the other hand, if thinking about your goal makes you feel good then that's a good indication that you believe that it's going to happen and you will be more likely to do what it's going to take to achieve your desired objective.

Of course, you need to think about goals that are realistic for you. For example, a goal to live until you are over a hundred years old is no longer unrealistic. It is estimated that there are approximately 200,000 centenarians in the world (those who have lived a century). In the United States alone according to the 2010 US Census Bureau, there were 53,364 people over 100 years old. If that is your goal you will want to remain healthy and active like Herman Goldman of New Jersey who turned 101 in august 2014 and still continues to drive himself to work four days per week to the same job he has had for the past 73 years at Capital Lighting in East Hanover. So, if living to be a centenarian is your goal you need think about what would motivate you to have this goal and what you are going to do to achieve it.

A goal to live a healthy life beyond your one hundredth birthday is no longer unrealistic.

If you tell yourself you want to be a sprinter in the Olympics and just thinking about that makes you depressed because you don't think that's going to happen, then maybe a better goal would be to run a half marathon by next year. A logical consequence of you starting to work towards the attainment of this goal would be incremental steps towards future lengthier runs. Your goal needs to be believable in order for you to feel good about it. If it's not or you don't feel good about that goal when you're reviewing it in your mind then you should consider simplifying it or change it to make it believable for you.

If you are interested in further readings related to this topic, we have provided some links at the end of this section.

Thirty Day Action Plan

Calculate your hip and waist ratios and again write that down on the downloadable form and at the end of this chapter. Then determine your Metabolic Type. You may also choose to find the Direct Labs in your area to complete your comprehensive wellness profile (www.directlabs.com). As we mentioned before, if there are any out-of-range scores on your blood work, you will obviously want to discuss the results with your family doctor. Finally, be diligent about following through on your 'Daily Thought Exercise'.

Remember that the thought exercise is simply thinking intently on a desired health and wellness goal. Where you want to see yourself going? Make sure it's believable and that you have a burning desire to make that happen. Of course, you can always adapt, modify or change your goals. That will likely be the case for most people. Thinking about and working towards an achievable goal will make you feel good and more likely to achieve that goal.

Chapter 3 - Nutrition and Exercise For Optimal Health

This chapter provides you with easy to follow strategies related to exercise and nutrition. We will give you an easy-to-follow work-out program that can be readily adapted to your level of fitness. The related exercise videos and hand-outs can readily be accessed online.

Introduction to Nutrition & Exercise Fundamentals

We are going to encourage you to move around, do some exercise and possibly even change the food in your refrigerator. To assist with the exercise portion of the chapter, we have hired a fitness guru to create a customized body weight fitness program that can readily be adapted to your particular level of fitness. This entire exercise program is available on video and can be accessed and downloaded to your home computer using the website link we provide to our readers.

The nutrition fundamentals part of the chapter aims to provide some basic background information and rationales as to food choices, what you may choose to add to your diet or to eliminate from your diet. We have provided a sample seven day diet and nutritional program for those individuals who feel ready to take on the challenge.

Introduction to Exercise

If you are somewhat of a novice to exercise and if you are not feeling particularly fit or maybe you haven't done a whole lot of stretch type exercises, then you may want to approach this exercise program on alternate days or perhaps three days a week to start. As your fitness level improves you can progressively build up the duration and difficulty of your workouts. On the other hand, if you are fairly active and physically fit, you can probably start with a six day a week program...work out six days then take one day to rest. The important thing to keep in mind is that every person should start at his or her own fitness level and incrementally add on a bit more each time.

If you notice that you're getting increasingly sorer and you find yourself doing less and less, then you're probably pushing yourself too much. So, that is when you may want to listen to your body and decrease your workout to fewer repetitions. We have a number of slides, print outs, and several different videos, including warm-ups and exercises that you can download to your own computer.

IT IS IMPORTANT TO LISTEN TO YOUR OWN BODY

Basic Exercise Program

Warm-Up Videos

There are two warm-up videos; the first video contains three exercises. The first exercise demonstrates how to do deep breathing to help oxygenate your blood. The other two exercises illustrate how to stretch and limber up your muscles and ligaments. The second warm-up video contains exercises that demonstrate several different types of stretches.

Crocodile Breathing

In this first video, we look at how to do proper breathing, specifically deep breathing. We refer to this deep breathing as crocodile breaths. This video demonstrates how to properly do this deep breathing. It's a good idea to do this particular exercise before you do your work out. It does several things. It gets your blood oxygenated, your nervous system prepped up and ready so that you are in the right space to begin the demonstrated exercises.

Crocodile Breathing 10-15 breaths

The first warm up portion is crocodile breathing. We just want to teach your body how to breath, getting your breaths set. Think about breathing into your nose, out through your nose, nice and controlled. Breath in your belly is if you're trying to fill a balloon and exhale through your nose. Think about a balloon deflating as you exhale. Do 10 breaths to start. You can work up to 15 once you're comfortable. Laying face down, hands on the forehead just relax. Breathing slowly through the nose filling up that belly and a brief slowly back out through the nose. Do 10 repetitions of this.

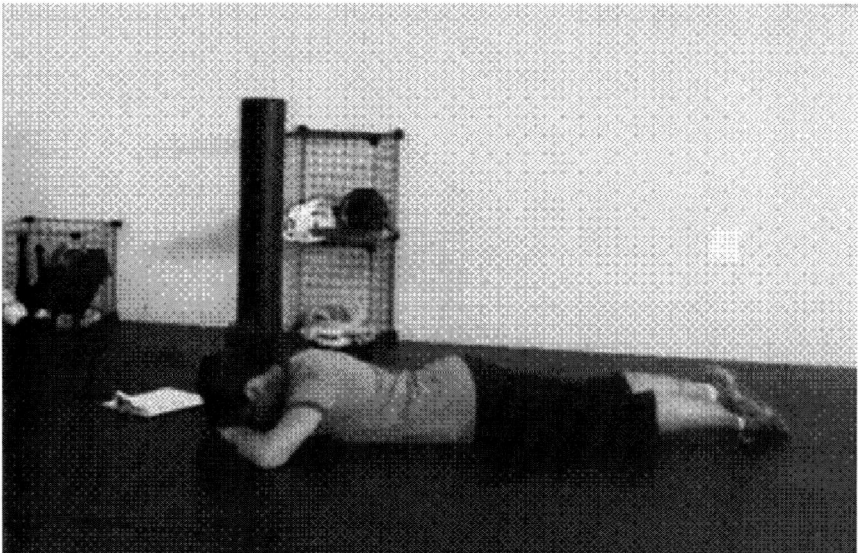

See the full video at http://youtu.be/5VKMJCydOGc

Walking/Jumping Jacks

Once you have completed your deep breathing warm ups, it's important to get the joints, ligaments and muscles warmed up. Engaging in brisk walking or doing jumping jacks or both are effective ways to get the body limbered up for the work-out exercises.

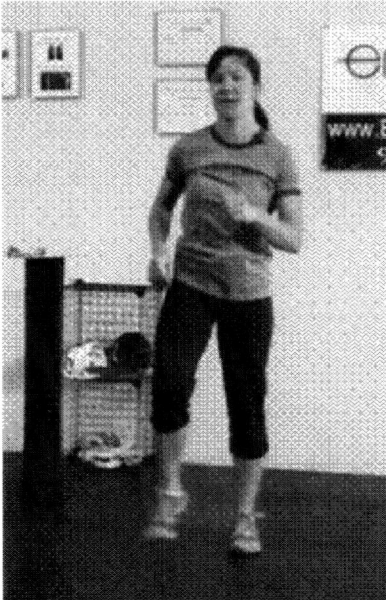

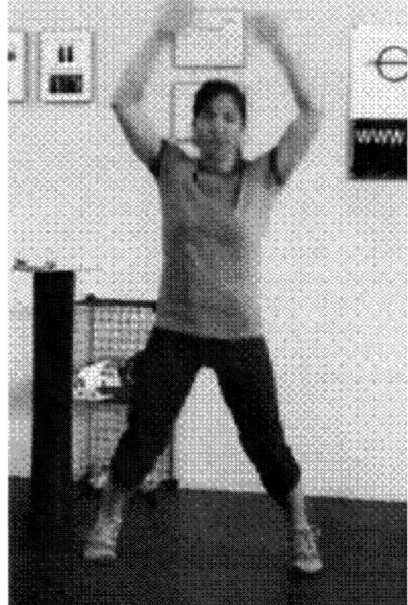

Foam Rolling

A foam roller is similar to what children use in the pool, but it's a little thicker and firmer. Utilizing the foam roller helps to stretch and condition your muscles. It is a great way to help push lactic acids from the muscles, to lengthen the muscles and possibly to work out some of those tight knots in there. It's like having a massage without the massage therapist. Time constraints may necessitate limiting the foam rolling to only a couple of times a week, but if you feel it's helpful, include it as a part of your warm-up program whenever you can. Again, the important thing is to listen to your body and follow through accordingly.

Remember to print out the warm-up exercises so you can use them in conjunction with the videos.

Foam Rolling: Glutes

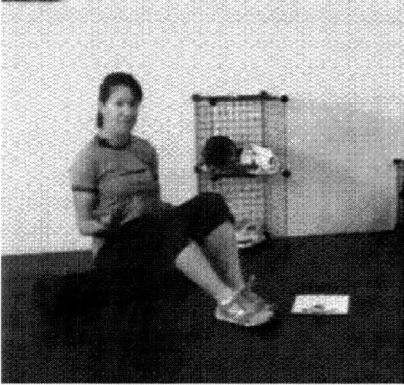

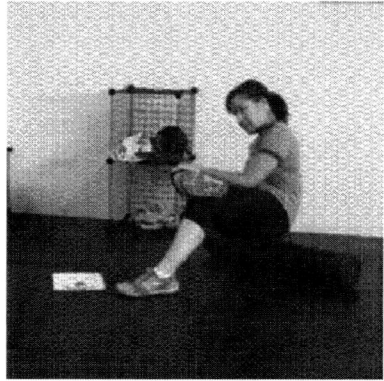

Foam Rolling: Upper Back

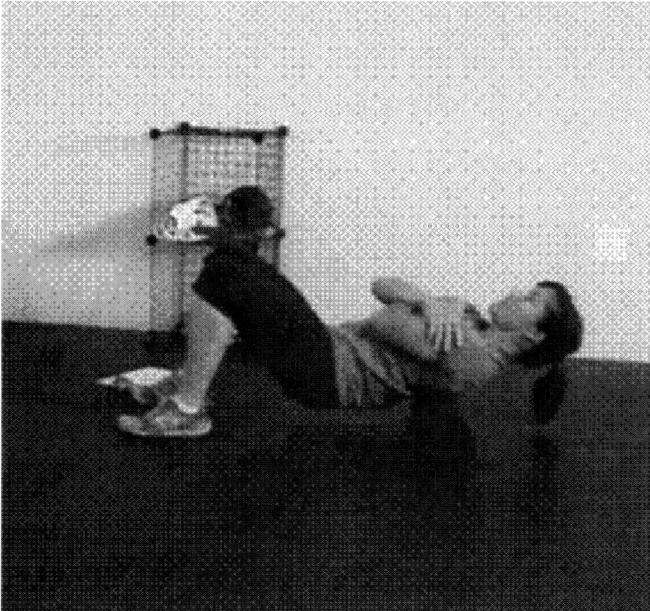

Foam Rolling: Lats

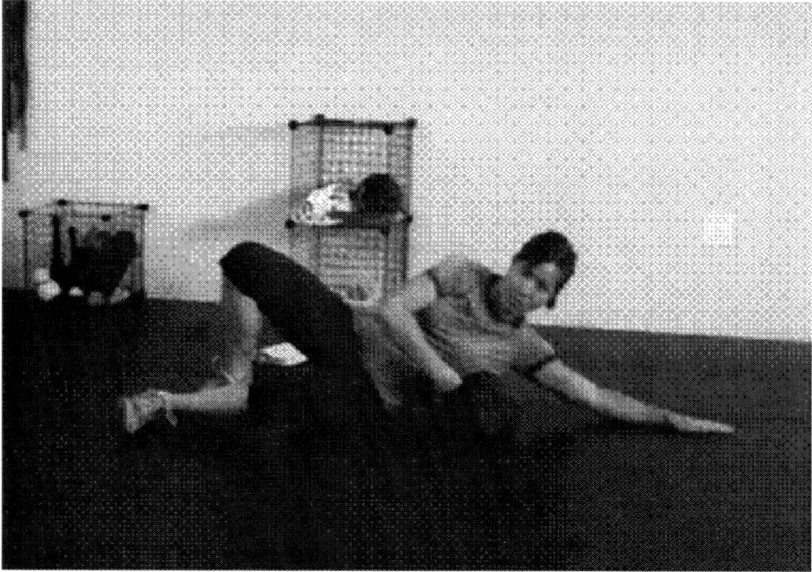

Foam Rolling: Quads

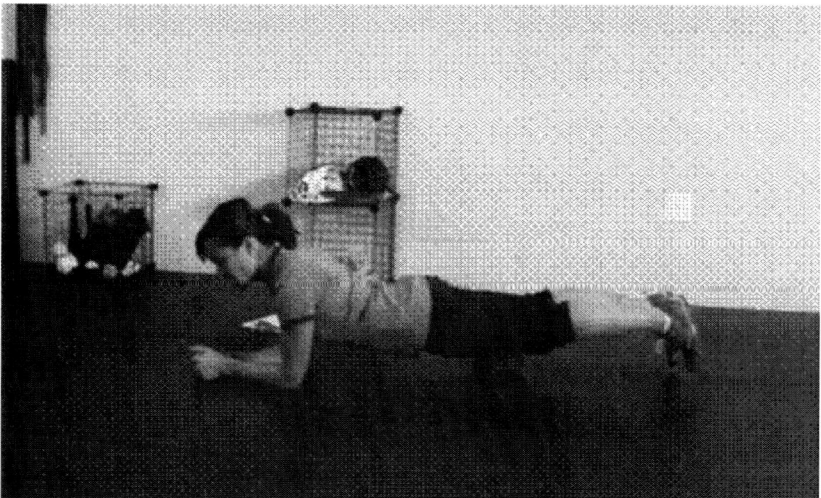

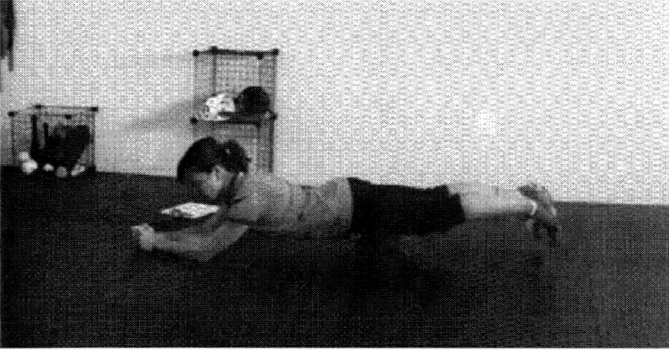

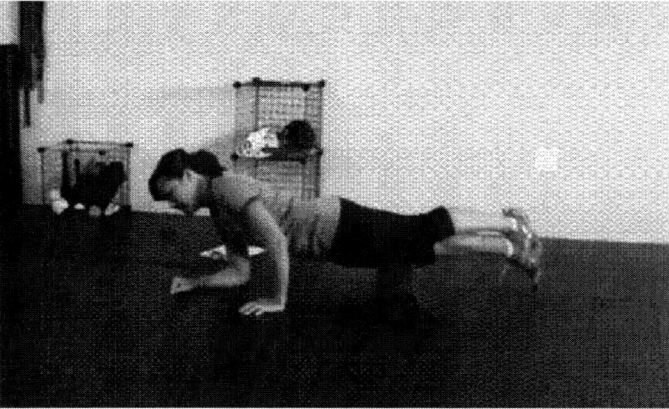

Foam Rolling: Inner Thigh

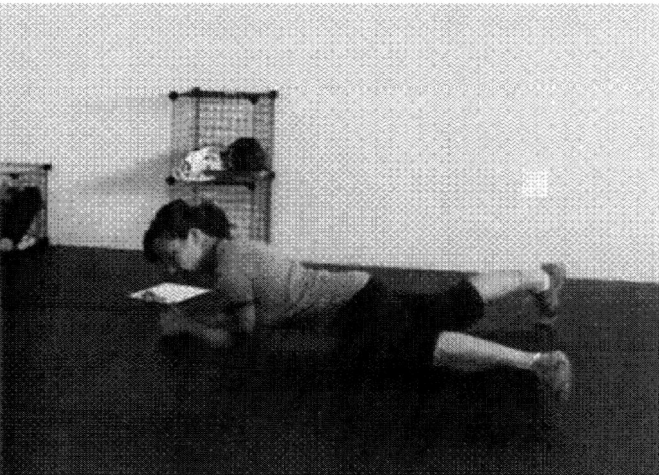

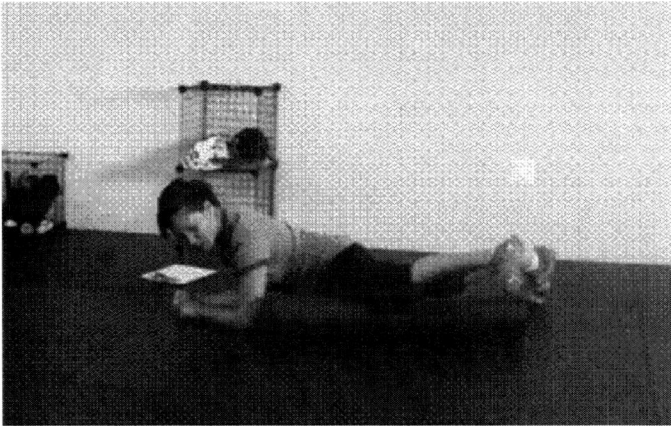

Warm-Up Video 2
See the full video at http://youtu.be/MzlsEaovdok

Stretches

In the first warm-up video we demonstrated exercises to stretch and limber up the muscles. The second video in the warm-up process focuses on several different types of stretches. It's important to stretch not only before a work out, but additionally after you complete each workout.

Stretches: Wall Slides

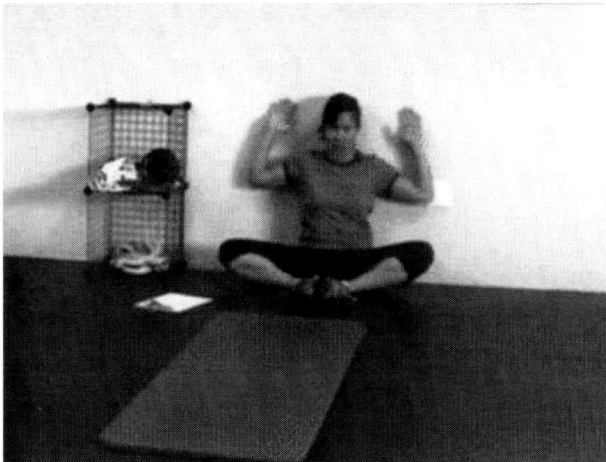

With wall slides we are correcting posture by placing our hips, back and head against the wall and slowly sliding our arms up the wall. If you feel pain or if your arms come off the wall you have reached your end or range of motion. Go slowly and enjoy the stretch.

Stretches: Hip Flexor

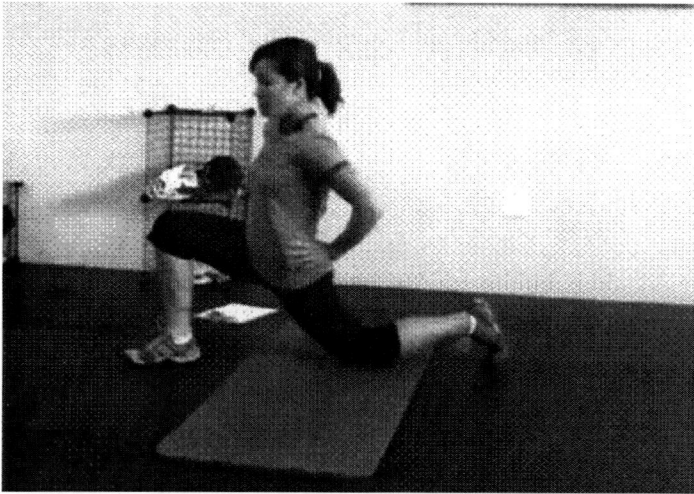

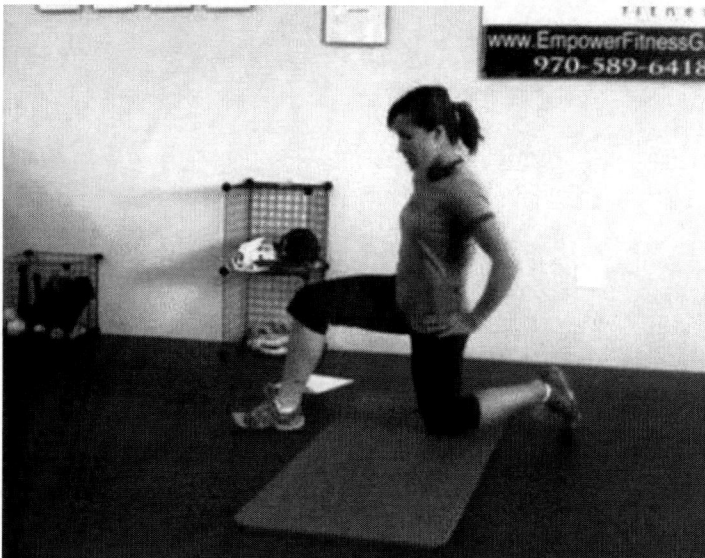

The hip flexor stretch is great for those who sit at a desk all day. The hip flexors shorten and can give us a lot of hip and low back pain. Follow the exercise instruction sheet.

Mobility

The next segment of the warm-up video focuses on mobility. These range of motion exercises take your joints and ligaments through their normal range of motion to help you to get an improved range of motion in some of the different joints. The key to this particular portion is slow and controlled movements. Make sure you are not over stretching or pushing it too far.

Mobility: 3-Way Neck

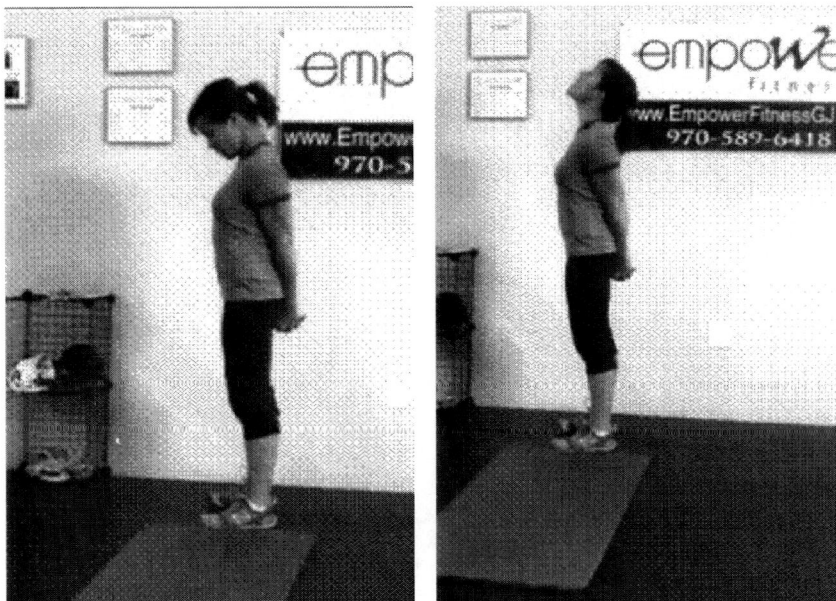

Clasp hand behind you, roll shoulder back and down, tuck chin and hold a few seconds, then look up and hold a few seconds. Helps correct poor "rolled" shoulders.

44

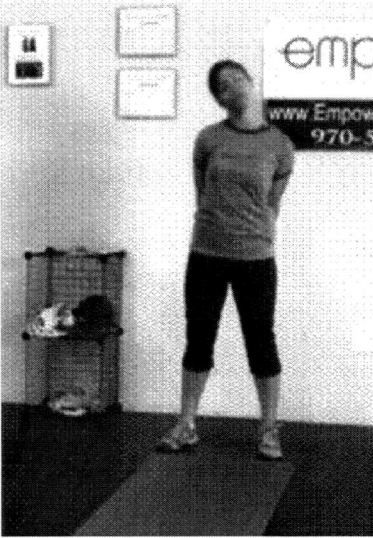

Same idea, this time tilting the head from side to side, holding several seconds each time.

Mobility: Seated T Spine Twist

Sit down cross legged, hands behind your head. Think tall. Chest open. Pull elbow back and you turn. Stay tall. Movement through thoracic spine. Five reps in each direction; ten total.

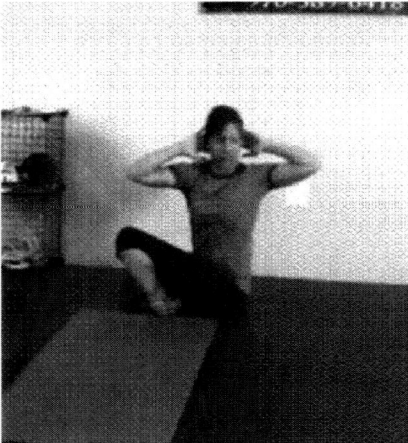

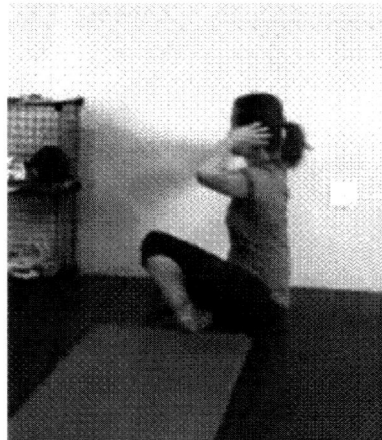

Mobility: Wrist Circles

Five to ten reps each way. Start by clasping your palms together. Rotate wrists in a circular movement, stretching out the wrists and forearm muscles.

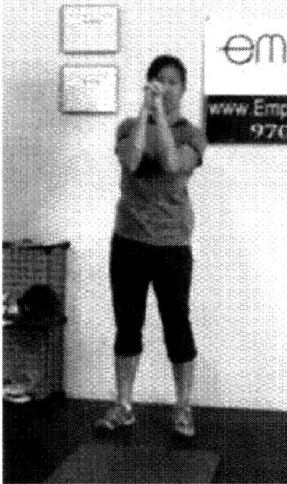

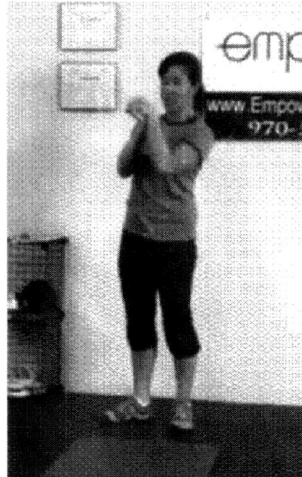

Mobility: Elbow Circles

Hands out, thumbs up, bring hands in and rotate down towards the floor bending the elbows. Do five rotations one way and five the reverse way.

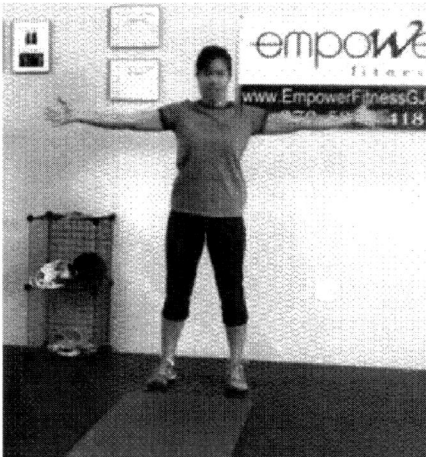

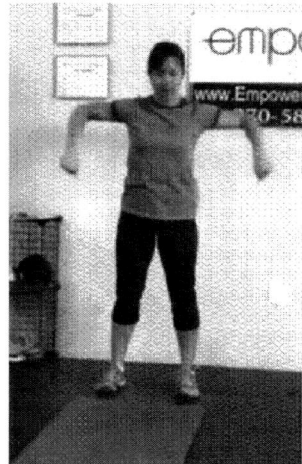

Mobility: Hula Hoop Circles

Feet shoulder width apart, start rotating hips around in a circle like you are spinning a hula hoop. Five in one direction, five in the opposite.

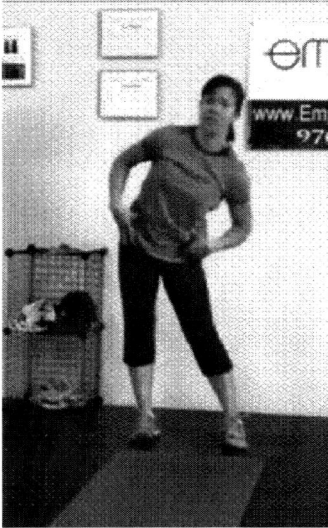

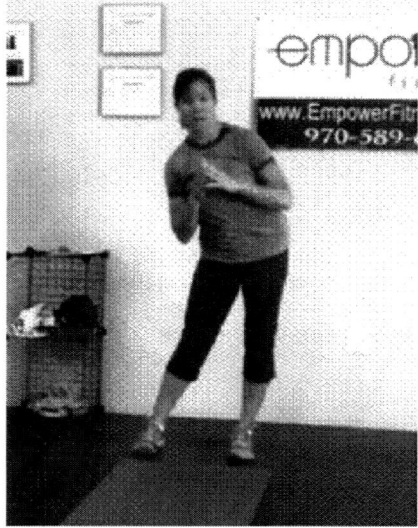

Mobility: Knee Circles

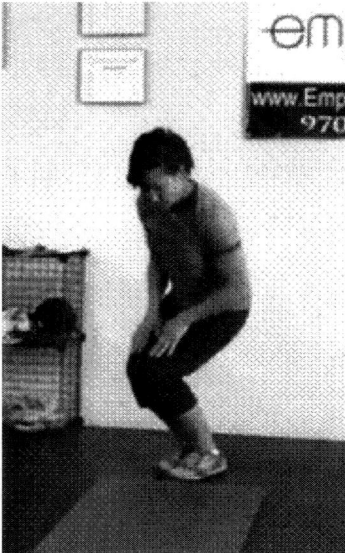

Start with your feet together and hand above knees. Similar movement as with the hula hoop, except the rotations happen at the knees and ankles.

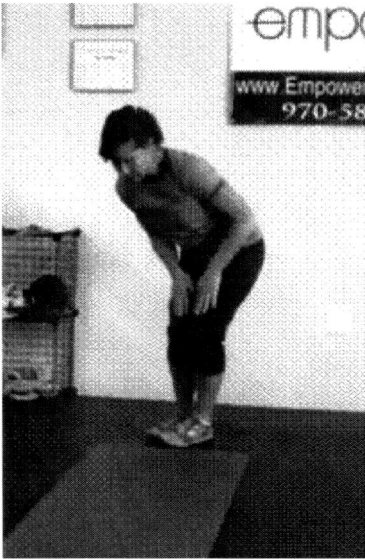

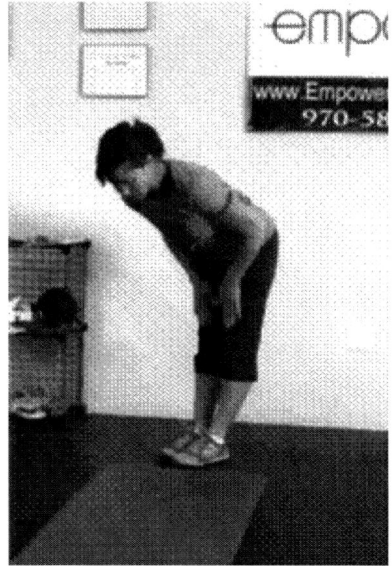

Mobility: Touch the Wall Deadlift

Standing up straight, arms out in front, "reach" forward as you bend the knees and jet your hips back while gently arching your back. 10 reps

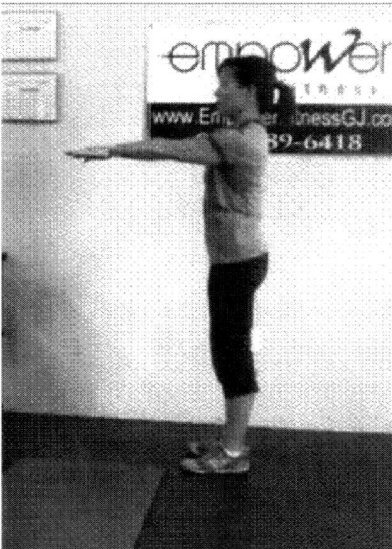

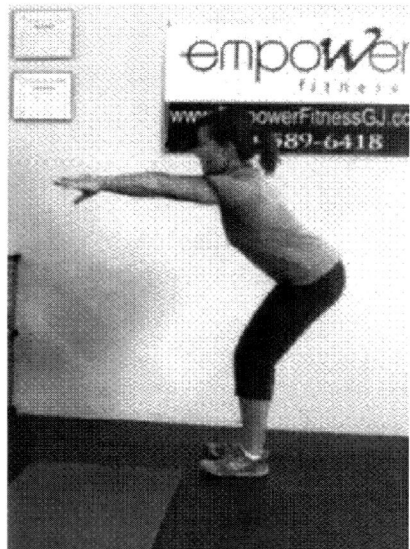

Correctives

The final segment of the warm up looks at corrective movements.

Corrective: Cook Hip Lift

This one helps engage the glutes. Start with one knee up and bend, hands on knee. The other heel is down. Drive the heel into the ground as you raise the hip up and hold for several seconds. 5 reps on each side.

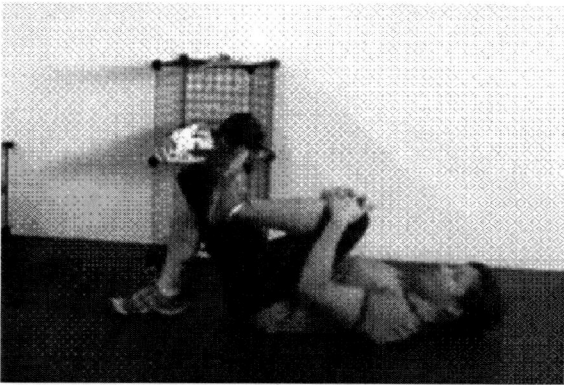

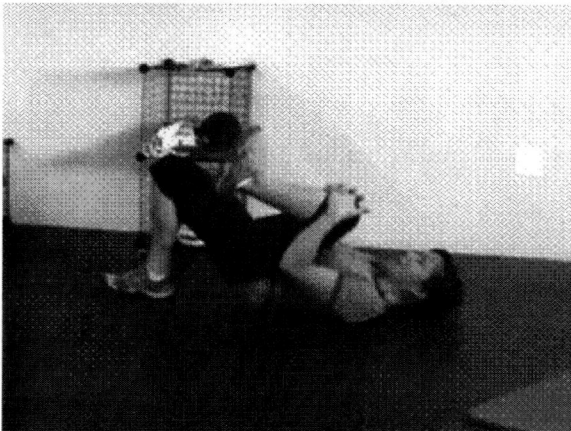

Exercise Videos

Once you have completed the warm-ups, you can move into the actual work out video.

Power and Core

The core is basically that area between the thoracic spine and the pelvis. It's the area where many people are somewhat de-conditioned. A de-conditioned core can predispose you to low back problems or increased susceptibility to back injuries, so it's very important when you're doing an exercise program to focus at least some segment of your workout on this critical area.

As you're going through the other exercises, make a point of activating the core as well. Regardless of how boring the power and core exercises may appear, it's an important part of the workout program, so try to make a point of not skipping over this segment.

See full video at http://youtu.be/Rhf6Jl3fvXk

1/4 Get Up

There will be three 1/4 Get Ups on each side. Don't let the simplicity of this core exercise fool you. Start by laying on your back, right knee bent, relax the other leg out to the side slightly, left arm out at the same angle, flat on the floor, right arm with a clenched fist pointing up towards the ceiling - start the core movement by raising the right fist toward the ceiling as you come up onto your left elbow and also leading with your stomach/core area, chest open and come completely up, left hand palm on the floor. Reverse the movement back down by relaxing and sinking the chest down slightly, move onto your left elbow while bringing the right fist down, using your core to lower you, lay back flat. Do three reps then switch sides.

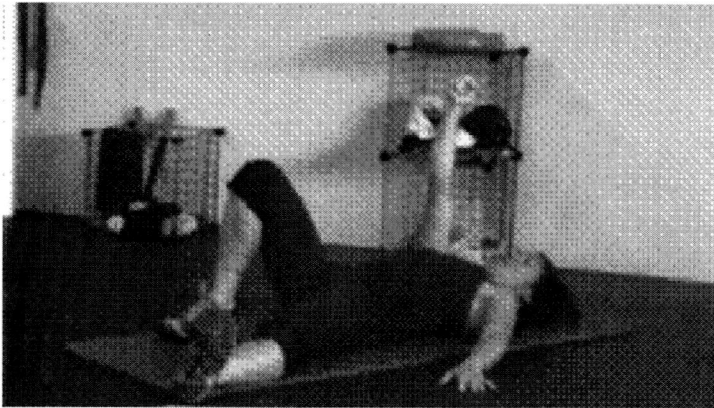

Flat Knee Raises

Start by laying flat on your back, bring the knees up into the chest, extend the legs up toward the ceiling, then lower back down and slightly tap the heels on the floor. Do five reps.

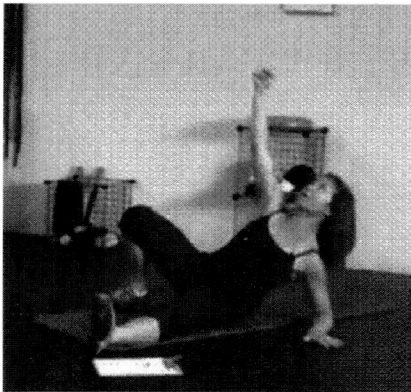

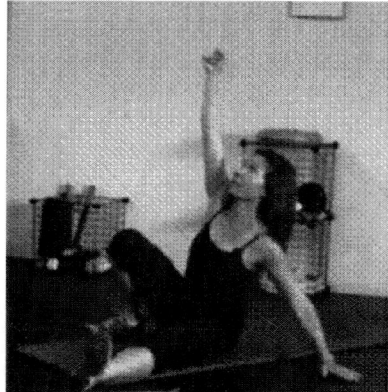

Referencing your Workout Handout which can be downloaded from this link: http://thewellnesssolution.co/wp-content/uploads/2012/11/Empower-BW.pdf

We will be doing two sets of the 1/4 Get up and Flat Knee Raise, alternating the two until you have done two sets of each.

Focus Circuit

The final component of your workout for your first week are the focus circuit exercises. These are exercises that work the muscles and get the heart rate up. After the first week, as your muscles and ligaments get used to these new movements and your overall conditioning improves, you should be ready to move on the secondary circuit part of the exercise program, but again it's important to listen to your body. Some of you might be able to do the secondary circuit the first week and others may need to wait a bit longer to add the secondary circuit to your workout. If you are feeling increasingly sore during the first week of your workout, you may want to decrease the number of repetitions.

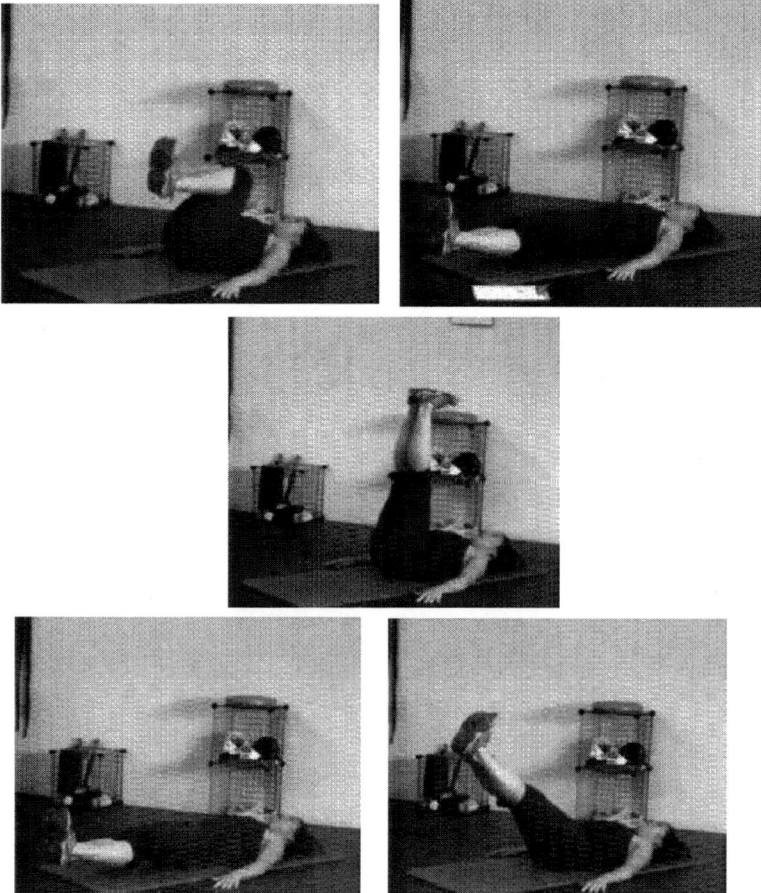

RKC Planks

These planks are a little different from others you may have done. Start with your feet together, thighs together, propped up on your elbows. Raise up onto your toes and elbows by squeezing your gluten and thighs together - holding for a five count. Lower back down till you are resting on your thighs and elbows. We will do three reps, two sets, alternating with other Focus Circuit exercises.

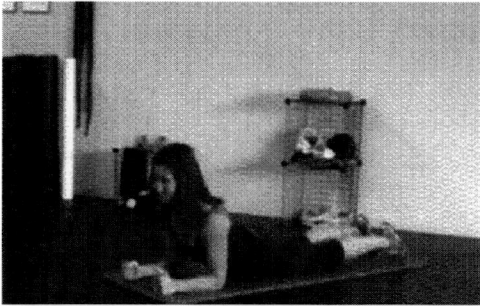

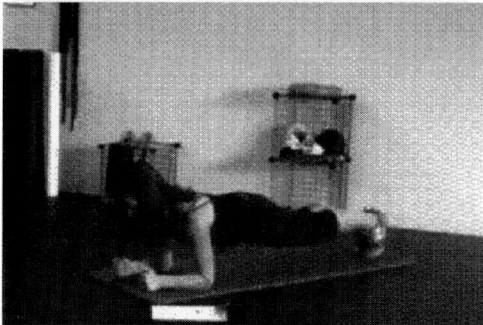

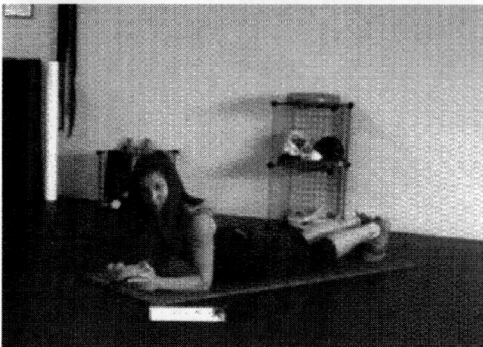

Glute Bridge

Laying on your back, feet shoulder width apart, contract the gluten and drive the core up flat in line with the knees and shoulders. Drive the heels and shoulders into the ground as the hips come up off the floor. We will do three reps, two sets alternating with the other exercises in this section.

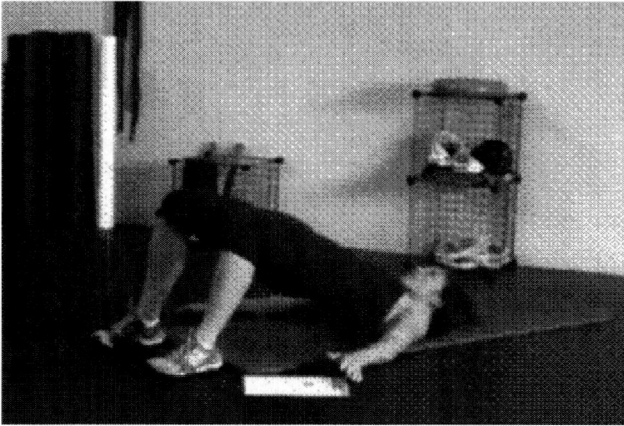

BW Squat

Start shoulder width apart, toes can be slightly pointed out. Drive your tail bone down towards the floor, then drive from the heel and come back up. We will do 10 reps and 2 sets, alternating with the other Focus Circuit exercises.

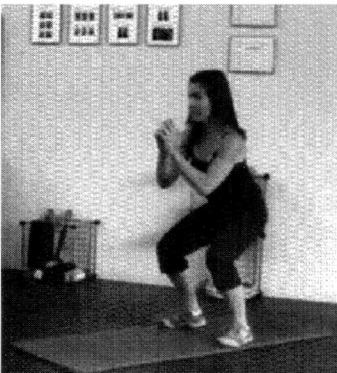

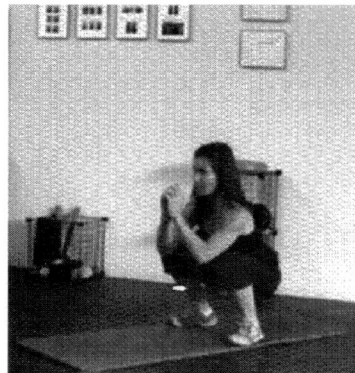

This ends the exercises for week 1. The Secondary Circuit exercises (Split Squat and Push Up) will be skipped this first week. They should be blacked out on your exercises sheet on the online handout, http://thewellnesssolution.co/wp-content/uploads/2012/11/Empower-BW.pdf

Secondary Circuit

Split Squat

Start feet a fair distance apart and lower down. Week 2 and beyond we will do eight reps, each leg, two sets alternating with the Push Ups.

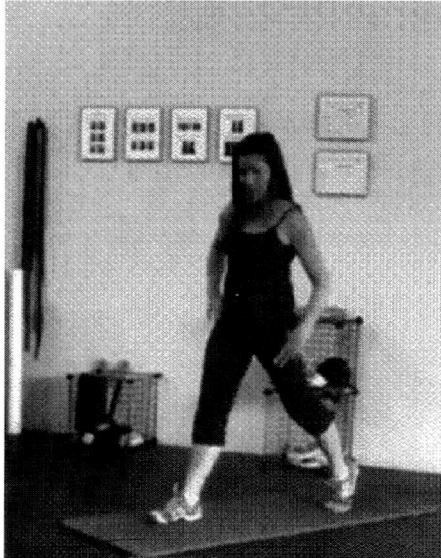

Push Up

These are your basic pushups. Start with hands shoulder width apart, up on your toes, legs apart. Go down to the ground keeping the back straight. Slightly touch and come back up. For those that can't do a normal push up, start in the same position, go down, and the get back up, drop to your knees and push back up, then get back into the starting position - palms flat on the floor and on your toes, repeat. We will do several of these (do what you are comfortable with, maybe start with three). We will alternate these with the Split Squat, two sets each.

Alternative Push Up (no girl pushups)

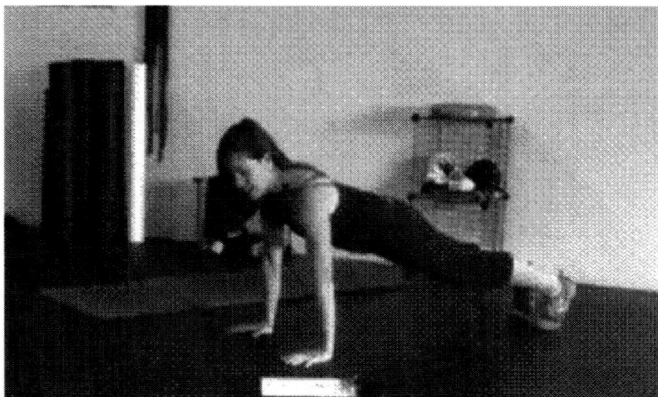

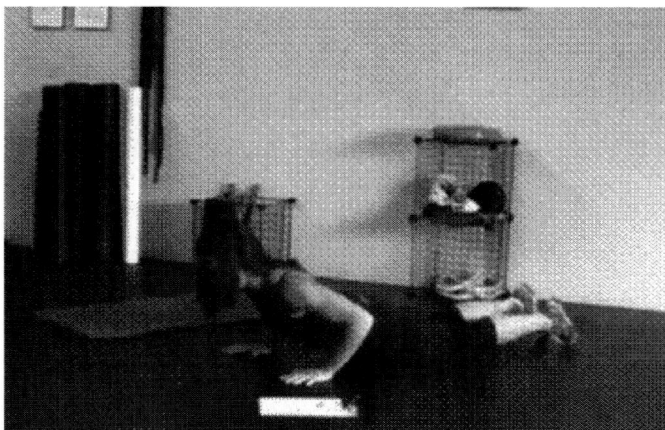

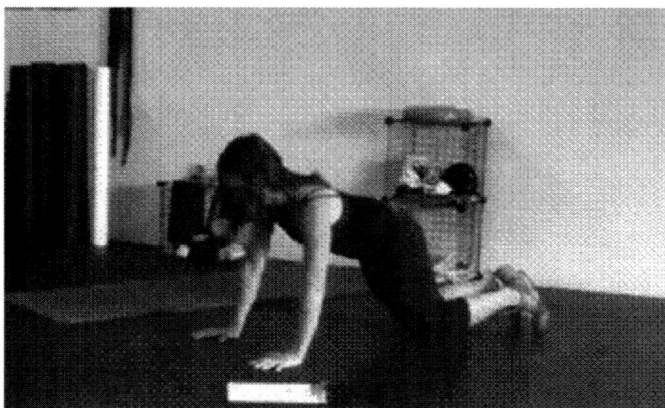

Intervals Video

Interval exercises are explosive repeats, basically 20 seconds of work, 40 seconds of rest. There are many different types of exercises that can be done during interval training. In the accompanying video, jump roping, jumping jacks, sprints and squats are demonstrated. The demonstrated interval exercises are intended for more advanced individuals who are well conditioned. For some of you, you may be ready for the interval exercises after you have completed the other workouts for a month or so, and others who already feel well conditioned, may be ready to add this component after the first week.

Once you are feeling well conditioned, you may choose to adjust your workout to better accommodate your daily schedule. For example, on days when you are pressed for time and simply don't have time to do the entire workout, you could go ahead and do the warm up video and then just jump right in to the intervals video. It is great way to get the blood flowing, to get the heart rate up and to speed up the fat burning process. Again, make sure that you are first fairly well conditioned. So, if on a particular day you are in a rush and simply don't have time to do a complete work out this may be an option for you, but again first make sure your body is sufficiently well conditioned.

See the full Intervals video at http://youtu.be/d2oOW-oETls

For intervals, we will be doing 20 seconds of work followed by 40 seconds of rest and we will do that six times - you can do a lot of different movements from jumping jacks to sprints, jump roping, etc. For the purpose of this chapter, we will have you do the Squat Matrix. Get a timer (phone, watch, etc.) and get into position for Body Weight Squats. At a fairly rapid pace, do squats for 20 seconds keeping good form.

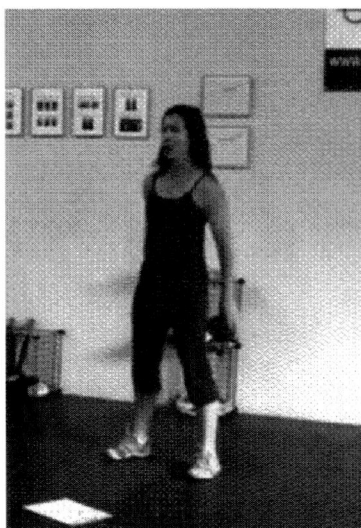

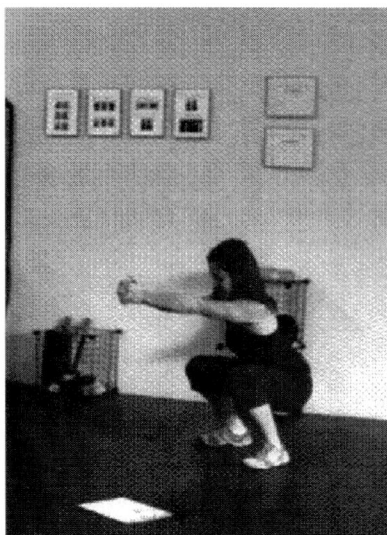

Rest for 40 seconds then do Squat Holds. Again, keep good form, hold the squat for 20 seconds, then rest for 40 seconds.

Next let's do speed squats with a jump. 20 seconds of work, 40 seconds of rest.

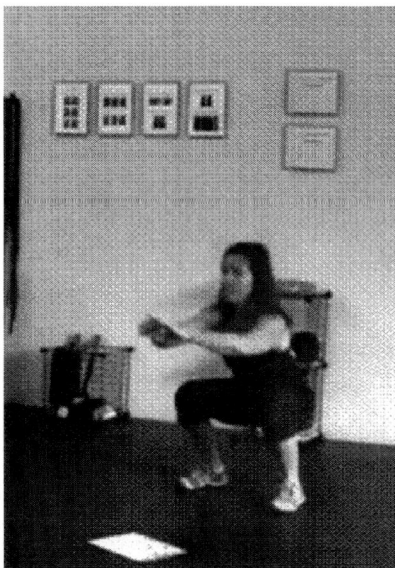

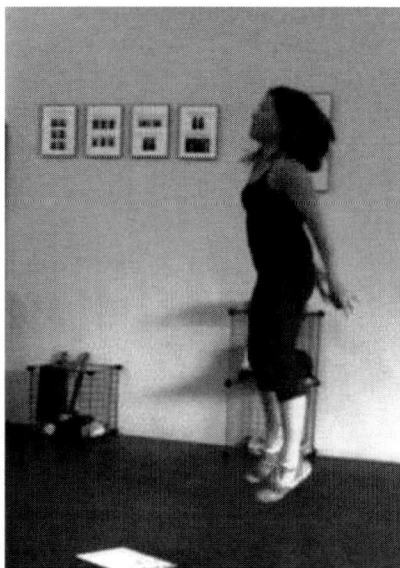

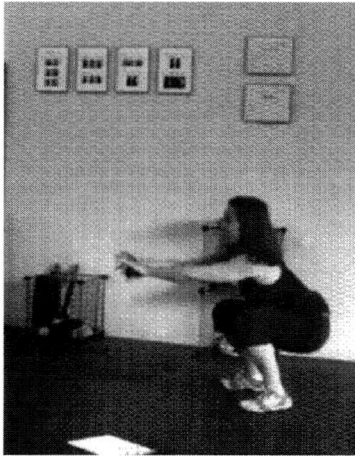

Now that you have done three intervals, we will repeat the first three to get our six intervals in. Repeat the body weight squats, speed squats with jump, and squat hold – two seconds of work, 40 seconds of rest.

Nutrition Fundamentals

The intent of this section is simply to give you some basic background information regarding foods you may consider adding to your diet or eliminating from your diet and a rationale as to why you may wish to consider making these changes.

Much has been written recently about eating foods that mimic as closely as possible the diets of our ancestors. So basically, what that looks like is eating all the lean meats, fruits, vegetables, nuts and seeds you want.

We will also look at some heavily lobbied foods and why eating these foods may create problems. Accompanying this chapter is a seven-day eating plan that you can choose to follow as is, or adapt to fit your particular lifestyle. This is something you can print out and start right away if you choose to.

We have left out two foods—wheat and dairy—that are considered healthy staples by a majority of the population. Although you may not want to eliminate these from your diet, you may want to consider reducing the amount or types of dairy and grains you consume. There is a considerable amount of recent research that suggests that excessive consumption of dairy and grains may create health issues. There are a number of different components of dairy and grains when eaten in excess that can predispose you to certain health problems.

People who are lactose intolerant will need to avoid dairy completely and similarly those individuals with gluten intolerance or allergies will need to stick to gluten-free products. For others, it's about keeping in mind that too much of anything can be harmful, so it's mainly about moderation. Also, understand that dairy and grains such as wheat are in the top 10 for common food allergies with dairy at number 1. (12) Overconsumption of these food products may have led to these allergies for many people.

Dairy

There is some research to suggest that the break-down of lactose in the gut from dairy may increase the risk for cataracts formation. (3, 4) So some individuals who have a family history of cataracts may want to investigate this further or discuss this with their health care provider. Over the years, numerous investigations related to the examination of possible causes of and cures for acne have been conducted. There is some evidence that can be drawn from this literature to suggest that dairy may impair iron and zinc abortion which can be a concern for acne-prone individuals. (5) Zinc helps the skin repair and heal itself so the ability to absorb zinc is important to skin health. If you are predisposed to acne and are consuming large quantities of dairy, you may want to re-visit this and adjust your diet accordingly. (6)

Also looking at dairy an interesting study came out back in 2007, a meta-analysis that looked at Parkinson's disease and they found that men that consumed the most dairy had an 80% increase in the risk of developing Parkinson's disease. (7) What the study didn't show was why. What is it about dairy consumption that causes that increased risk? Noticing that is definitely a concern. More studies need to be done to find out exactly what's happening to increase that risk, but obviously that's a concern. These above stated findings were further supported by an additional study called the Honolulu Heart Study which examined 7,504 men. These men were followed for some 30 years for any development of Parkinson's Disease. The study showed that there was a 2.3 times greater occurrence of Parkinson's Disease in those men that drank the most milk compared to those who abstained from milk. (8) Additional studies have found similar this same link. (10)

There are some studies to suggest that dairy may increase mucous production for some individuals and predispose them to ear aches, infections and asthma. So again, this may be something to consider. (11)

There are a number of studies looking at the possible connection between babies and colic and cow's milk. In the early days of infant formula formation cow's milk was used as the base in the composition of the formula. It was observed that if the baby was taken off the formula, the colic would clear up. Now you cannot buy infant formula with cow's milk as the base because of the assumed correlation between cow's milk and colic.

Today breast milk is recommended as the healthiest option for infants to bolster the child's immune system and to counter the development of possible allergies. A recent study suggests that even mothers drinking cow's milk could possibly cause colic in their babies. It is postulated that there may be something that is passing through the mother's milk to the infant that may cause the colic because when the mother was taken off the milk the colic cleared up. When the mother started consuming milk again, the colic come back again. (13)

There appears to be a high incidence of childhood allergic reactions to milk. Although children appear to grow out of the milk allergy by the age of three or four, there is concern that there may be a possible link between the children who as infants and toddlers may have had allergic reactions to milk and possible future allergic reactions to certain foods in later years. Is there something about drinking milk early that seems to change how the immune system responds to food? This possible link would have to be examined with further research.

Another concern is that dairy contains bovine estrogen. High dosages of estrogen have been associated with higher risks of prostate cancer, breast cancer and even ovarian cancer. However, consensus as to how much is too much is still under debate. (14,15,16, 17, 18, 19)

There is also a growing body of evidence that excessive calcium intake such as that from dairy and supplemental calcium is associated with a significantly increased risk of heart attacks and sudden death. These findings were reported in a 2010 meta-analysis published in the British Journal of Medicine by researchers from the University of Auckland. Their analysis looked at 26 separate studies and involved over 20,000 individuals. (20) Other research suggests that high blood levels of calcium are possibly involved in the development of atherosclerosis (clogged arteries) (21) because too much calcium may promote the formation and fragility of the plaques which block our arteries.

At some point in the past, it was thought that dairy raised blood sugar levels, but that was proven to be a false assumption since the glycemic index was developed and founds that dairy had low glycemic responses. (22) However, dairy does appear to significantly raise insulin levels. The problem with high levels of blood insulin is the risk of developing insulin resistance, which is the precursor to metabolic syndrome and diabetes. (23, 24, 25, 26, 27, 28)

There also appears to be a correlation with acne and dairy consumption as well. (29, 30, 31, 32, 33, 34, 35, 36) It may be in part because as we know dairy spikes blood insulin levels, and we know that high insulin levels slows down the sloughing off of your skin cells and that in conjunction with the reduced zinc absorption issue may lead to acne. (29) Some researchers also feel that dairy in combination with a diet high in refined carbs may cause a hormone cascade effect that along with elevated insulin leads to acne. While the jury is still out on how dairy contributes to acne, the data is clear that if you take individuals with acne off of dairy for thirty days their acne either clears up or vastly improves.

Another concern related to dairy that has surfaced more recently is that dairy contains an insulin-like growth factor or IGF-1. We know that IGF-1 promotes cell growth and proliferation, both of healthy cells and cancer cells (37, 38) and drinking milk has been shown to raise IGF-1 levels in the blood. (39) It appears to readily cross the gut into the blood stream. Studies show that high IGF-1 increases the risk of cancer growth especially prostate and breast (40, 41) and milk drinking also seems to increase in general the risk of ovarian cancer. (42, 43)

In a way, cow's milk is basically just filtered cow's blood, so all the hormones, the pesticides, the proteins, everything that is in the cow's blood minus the red and white blood cells is in their milk, so with that you're getting a lot of those constituents. In general, milk is designed for fattening up the calf. When humans consume an excess of this particular food group over a length of time all those different hormones can stimulate the body in a lot of different ways, ways that we probably don't even understand. So again, the point here is simply to exercise moderation. A little bit is probably okay, but drinking an excess may be problematic as we have seen.

Grains

Over the years, we have heard over and over that we need to consume grains, especially whole wheat and other whole grains because they are a good source of fiber. However, when you compare grains to other things such as fruits and vegetables they are lightweights when it comes to fiber. Also with grain consumption you are going to be ingesting a lot of other constituents of grains which are considered anti-nutrients such as phytate and glutens and perhaps preservatives as well. In general, phytate is considered an anti-nutrient. It has a binding effect to minerals so it not only binds together minerals that come with the grain but also other minerals in your gut as well.

So, wheat may be a good source of these minerals, but when you have phytate in the grain, it binds the minerals together and renders them unavailable for absorption. Consequently, you're not benefitting from these minerals in the grains. There is also evidence to suggest that grains, particularly wheat may impair vitamin D metabolism. Also, there is some concern that grains may increase susceptibility to inflammation because grains can make your body more acidic. The issue with acidity is the buffering effect your body has to go through, so it is going to be robbing certain minerals from your bone to buffer that acid in your blood. Therefore, over a long period of time high consumption of grains could predispose you to osteopenia, osteoporosis or other bone disorders.

Gluten, an anti-nutrient in grains, especially wheat can be concerning for some, particularly for those individuals with Celiac disease and gluten sensitivity. Gluten is that part in grains that makes dough pliable and stretchy and it gives the texture and softness so many have learned to love about breads. Unfortunately, the problem with gluten is that for a lot of individuals, it's an irritant to their gut and over time for some it may develop into Celiac Disease.

Facilitated by social media, we are learning that many more people than we originally thought either have or think they have Celiac Disease. The last estimate was one in a hundred people in the US. (44) That works out to approximately 2.3 million Americans who have or claim to have Celiac Disease...and that is a lot of people. Unfortunately, a significant number of individuals with Celiac Disease do not have gut symptoms but instead have other symptoms like ataxia, joint pain, migraines et cetera. So, they end up being misdiagnosed for years and their condition can worsen.

Some individuals who do not have Celiac Disease might still find that gluten consumption has an underlying effect on their gut health. This in turn could make them more prone to leaky gut. So, some people who do not have the serious immune responses and reactions experienced by those with Celiac Disease could still have an underlying response which over the long term could create serious complications because of their lack of awareness of the issue and failure to take corrective measures. There is a concern that with a leaky gut large proteins and molecules can pass right into the blood stream which can create a stronger response in the immune system and that can lead to other types of autoimmune diseases as well.

Diagnosing a gluten allergy can be a complex task because you can experience symptoms associated with a number of different health conditions or diseases, yet the primary root of these different health conditions might all be stemming from a gluten issue or a grain consumption issue. So, it can get very confusing particularly if your family physician is just looking at the symptom or just treating the symptom and not looking at the underlying cause. Perhaps this is why so many people go undiagnosed.

The symptoms of Celiac Disease, in and of itself, are broad. Some people don't even have digestive type symptoms. They might simply have swollen joints. The symptoms don't always have to be correlated to just the digestive issues. Even with gluten intolerance in general, many people may have some level of gluten intolerance because it is an anti-nutrient. Their symptoms could range from depression, anxiety, headaches or migraines to swollen joints and muscles.

So, instead of initially trying to do a lot of different testing to determine a single root cause, it may be a simpler option to first attempt an elimination diet. Try to avoid grains for thirty days and see how good you feel. It is remarkable how much better people can feel by just eliminating gluten containing grains and packaged foods for as little as thirty days.

We have noticed in our practice that if we can get someone to commit to getting off grains for thirty days their headaches and migraines often clear up and they almost always lose weight. Of course, a lot of that is going to be water weight because of the inflammation, as well as the weight from eating less carbohydrates, but additionally just getting off of grains will help stabilize blood sugars as well.

Two pieces of whole grain bread has the same insulin response as a tablespoon of sugar even though breads have added fiber. So again, taking someone off of sugar can have similar results as taking someone off of grains. You will naturally lose weight and feel better. In all likelihood, your joints will feel better and your blood acid will stabilize which in turn will decrease inflammation. For those of you who are somewhat skeptical about this, we challenge you to try going without grains for thirty days. You may be pleasantly surprised by how good you feel.

Eating Healthy Simplified Whole Foods

Over the years there have been numerous diets claiming their health benefits and potential to cure illnesses. One such widely publicized nutritional regimen was the Macro Diet. This diet was popularized by a physician who claims he was cured of cancer by following it. He was featured in a *Life Magazine* article titled "Physician Heal Thy Self."

More recently, much has been written about mimicking a diet similar to that of our ancestors. Books such as *The Paleo Diet* by Loren Cordain, advocating a return to the diets followed by the hunter-gatherer cultures and the *Wheat Belly* by Dr. William Davis, advocating gluten and wheat free diets have proven to be best sellers. Cordain contends that our ancestors didn't have degenerative diseases, heart attacks, stroke, cancer or osteoporosis and that as a whole they were much healthier than we are today because their diet consisted mainly of what they could pick out of the ground or shoot with a bow and arrow, so most of their meat was healthy, wild meat. This Paleo diet contained no dairy, grains or legumes such as green and pinto beans and obviously no processed foods.

Of course, in today's world following such a diet would be a major challenge. Additionally, we are now facing numerous challenges that were non-issues for our ancestors such as toxins and pesticides in the soil, air and water pollution, preservatives and genetic modification of our foods to name just a few of these. It appears that every day yet another human created food related issue is added to the list of concerns.

As mentioned earlier, following a hunter-gatherer, dairy and wheat-free diet could be a challenge and for many may not be an option they are prepared to choose. Also, the dairy and wheat available today is very different from that consumed in the past. Most dairy and wheat products today have been processed and contain various additives or preservatives. So, trying to mimic the diet of the hunter-gathers or even of our ancestors from a couple of thousand years ago can present a difficult challenge.

However, by choosing to eat basic non-processed, non-GMO modified, locally-grown, organic foods, cutting back on grains and dairy, and by following a diet that simulates as much as possible our early ancestors will undoubtedly make one a healthier person. We appreciate that eating meats or cutting out grains are not realistic options for many for a variety of reasons. Financial and time constraints, one's beliefs, values and cultural backgrounds often play important roles in decisions related to what we should eat and even how the food should be processed and eaten.

So, we are not saying that you should not be drinking milk at all or that you should not consume any products made with grains. Rather, the take-home message here is that simply by adding a few good things to your diet and eliminating some bad things and as much as possible selecting foods that our genes were designed to accommodate make us healthier.

The important point here is to just keep it simple and slowly start to clean up the diet. What we want to encourage is for you to start to make some small changes to healthier choices. Many of you may already have made those healthy choices, others may be at the early stages of making more healthy choices and for a few of you this may seem somewhat radical and overwhelming. So where do you start if this information is all brand new to you? You simply start from where ever you are at by just making small changes. Start by adding a few healthy things to your diet rather than trying to eliminate everything you're used to.

An elimination diet can be a problem because it can be difficult to break a habit or to change eating habits you may have been used to since you were a child. For example, if you're used to drinking a pot of coffee a day and then you just try to quit cold turkey but you've not replaced it with anything else, that may be very difficult so you may be better off to simply tell yourself that you will drink a glass of water for every cup of coffee you drink. By doing this it is likely that you will automatically start cutting back on your coffee consumption.

You may after a period of time get to a point where you are not drinking that much coffee anymore and instead you are drinking a lot more water. So, by adding good things to your diet, the bad things start to taper down. The same rational applies with soda. If you drink a six pack of soda a day, make a decision to drink a glass of water for every soda you consume.

You may find that after a while you might get to a place where you just start to crave that water. We have patients who say that they don't drink any water at all so we suggest to them that they try start by drinking small quantities of water and slowly and incrementally increase the amount. Over a period of time their body will start to crave water because it's getting something that it needs and once your body starts to crave the good things often those bad things start fall away on their own.

Thirty Day Action Plan

In conjunction with this chapter, we provide you with a seven- day sample healthy eating plan that you can download and print, at http://thewellnesssolution.co/wp-content/uploads/2012/11/7-day-healthy-eating-plan.pdf

This seven-day diet is a sample of what good healthy eating would look like. All the recipes are included for all the different items on that plan. This would be good for someone who is ready to make some pretty big changes.

Now granted, you might have a day a week where you eat a pizza or you have a soda or two a week. Again, what you do most of the time will dictate your overall health. It is not what you do every once in a while. So, this sample eating plan is simply an example of what super clean eating would look like.

We have several additional downloads available with this chapter. Nutrition Fundamentals outlines the foods that we are designed to eat and the foods that may be troublesome. These are at http://thewellnesssolution.co/wp-content/uploads/2012/11/Nutrition-Fundamentals.pdf

We have a cook book that is chock full of good recipes if you want to continue this type of diet or variations of it. Download it from http://thewellnesssolution.co/wp-content/uploads/2014/12/TWS-Healthy-Recipe-Book.pdf

Further Readings

For those of you who want to do some further reading on related topics, we suggest *The Paleo Diet* by Loren Cordain. This book talks about hunter-gatherer cultures and their diets and recommends foods for individuals wanting to follow this Paleo diet. The web site is http://thepaleodiet.com/

Wheat Belly by Dr. William Davis is another best-selling book. That web site is http://www.wheatbellyblog.com/. It discusses issues related to gluten, wheat and grains in general and how wheat and grain production and composition has changed over the centuries.

We also like *Grain Brain* by Dr. Perlmutter, who explains how carbs are destroying our brains. And not just unhealthy carbs, but even healthy ones like whole grains can cause dementia, ADHD, anxiety, chronic headaches, depression, and much more. The web site is http://www.drperlmutter.com/about/grain-brain-by-david-perlmutter/

Two additional resources you can purchase at Amazon are: *Perfect Health Diet* by Paul and Shou-Ching Jaminet (http://www. amazon.com/Perfect-Health-Diet-Regain-weight/dp/1451699158) and *Health at 100* by John Robbins (http://www.amazon.com/Hea lthy-100-Scientifically-Healthiest-Longest-Lived/dp/0345490118)

Chapter References:

1. http://www.direct-ms.org/pdf/EvolutionPaleolithic/Cereal%20Sword.pdf

2. https://s3.amazonaws.com/paleodietev02/research/Human+Diet+Its+Origins+and+ Evolution+The+Paleo+Diet.pdf

3. Couet C, Jan P, Debry G. Lactose and cataract in humans: a review. J Am Coll Nutr 1991;10:79-86.

4. http://thepaleodiet.com/dairy-milking-worth/

5. Castillo-Duran C, Solomons NW. Studies on the bioavailability of zinc in humans. IX. Interaction of beef-zinc with iron, calcium and lactose. Nutr Res 1991;11:429-38.

6. Cordain L, Lindeberg S, Hurtado M, Hill K, Eaton SB, Brand-Miller J. Acne vulgaris: a disease of Western civilization. Arch Dermatol. 2002 Dec;138(12):1584-90. http://thepaleodiet.com/research-about-the-paleo-diet/#2002

7. Chen H, O'Reilly E, McCullough ML, Rodriguez C, Schwarzschild MA, Calle EE, Thun MJ, Ascherio A. Consumption

of dairy products and risk of Parkinson's disease. Am J Epidemiol. 2007 May 1;165(9):998-1006.

8. Park M, Ross GW, Petrovitch H, White LR, Masaki KH, Nelson JS, Tanner CM, Curb JD, Blanchette PL, Abbott RD. Consumption of milk and calcium in midlife and the future risk of Parkinson disease. Neurology. 2005 Mar 22;64(6):1047-51

9. Park M, Ross GW, Petrovitch H, White LR, Masaki KH, Nelson JS, Tanner CM, Curb JD, Blanchette PL, Abbott RD. Consumption of milk and calcium in midlife and the future risk of Parkinson disease. Neurology. 2005 Mar 22;64(6):1047-51

10. Wilhelm KR, Yanamandra K, Gruden MA, Zamotin V, Malisauskas M, Casaite V, Darinskas A, Forsgren L, Morozova-Roche LA. Immune reactivity towards insulin, its amyloid and protein S100B in blood sera of Parkinson's disease patients. Eur J Neurol. 2007 Mar;14(3):327-34.

11. Bartley J, McGlashan SR.Does milk increase mucus production? Med Hypotheses. 2010 Apr;74(4):732-4.

12. National Institute of Allergy and Infectious Diseases (July 2004). "NIH Publication No. 04-5518: Food Allergy: An Overview.

13. Clyne, P.S., Kulczycki, A. Human breast milk contains bovine IgG. Relationship to Infant Colic? Pediatrics. 1992; 87: 439-444.

14. Gao X, LaValley MP, Tucker KL. Prospective studies of dairy product and calcium intakes and prostate cancer risk: a meta-analysis. J Natl Cancer Inst. 2005 Dec 7;97(23):1768-77.

15. Kurahashi N, Inoue M, Iwasaki M, et al. Dairy product, saturated fatty acid, and calcium intake and prostate cancer in a prospective cohort of Japanese men. Cancer Epidemiol Biomarkers Prev. 2008 Apr;17(4):930-7.

16. Qin LQ, Xu JY, Wang PY, Tong J, Hoshi K. Milk consumption is a risk factor for prostate cancer in Western countries: evidence from cohort studies. Asia Pac J Clin Nutr. 2007;16(3):467-76.

17. Qin LQ, Xu JY, Wang PY, Kaneko T, Hoshi K, Sato A. Milk consumption is a risk factor for prostate cancer: meta-analysis of case-control studies. Nutr Cancer. 2004;48(1):22-7

18. Rohrmann S, Platz EA, Kavanaugh CJ, et al. Meat and dairy consumption and subsequent risk of prostate cancer in a US cohort study. Cancer Causes Control. 2007 Feb;18(1):41-50.

19. Zucker GM, Clayman CB. Landmark perspective: Bertram W. Sippy and ulcer disease therapy. JAMA. 1983 Oct 28;250(16):2198-202.

20. Bolland MJ, Avenell A, Baron JA, Grey A, MacLennan GS, Gamble GD, Reid IR. Effect of calcium supplements on risk of myocardial infarction and cardiovascular events: meta-analysis. BMJ. 2010 Jul 29;341:c3691

21. Reid IR, Bolland MJ, Grey A. Does calcium supplementation increase cardiovascular risk? Clin Endocrinol (Oxf). 2010 Dec;73(6):689-95.

22. Foster-Powell K, Holt SH, Brand-Miller JC. International table of glycemic index and glycemic load values: 2002. Am J Clin Nutr. 2002 Jul;76(1):5-56.

23. Gannon MC, Nuttall FQ, Krezowski PA, Billington CJ, Parker S. The serum insulin and plasma glucose responses to milk and fruit products in type 2 (non-insulin-dependent) diabetic patients. Diabetologia. 1986 Nov;29(11):784-91.

24. Holt SH Miller JC, Petocz P. An insulin index of foods: the insulin demand generated by 1000-kJ portions of common foods. Am J Clin Nutr. 1997 Nov;66(5):1264-76

25. Hoyt G, Hickey MS, Cordain, L. Dissociation of the glycaemic and insulinaemic responses to whole and skimmed milk. Br J Nutr. 2005 Feb;93(2):175-7

26. Ostman EM, Liljeberg Elmståhl HG, Björck IM. Inconsistency between glycemic and insulinemic responses to regular and fermented milk products. Am J Clin Nutr 2001;74:96 –100.

27. Liljeberg Elmstahl H & Bjorck I. Milk as a supplement to mixed meals may elevate postprandial insulinaemia. Eur J Clin Nutr 2001; 55:994–999.

28. Hoppe C, Mølgaard C, Vaag A, Barkholt V, Michaelsen KF. High intakes of milk, but not meat increase s-insulin and insulin resistance in 8-year-old boys. Eur J Clin Nutr. 2005 Mar;59(3):393-8

29. Cordain L, Lindeberg S, Hurtado M, Hill K, Eaton SB, Brand-Miller J. Acne vulgaris: a disease of Western civilization. Arch Dermatol. 2002 Dec;138(12):1584-90.
http://thepaleodiet.com/research-about-the-paleo-diet/#2002

30. Cordain L. Implications for the role of diet in acne. Semin Cutan Med Surg. 2005 Jun;24(2):84-91
http://thepaleodiet.com/research-about-the-paleo-diet/#2005

31. Adebamowo, C.A. Spiegelman D, Danby FW, Frazier AL, Willett WC, Holmes MD. High school dietary dairy intake and teenage acne. J Am Acad Dermatol; 52(2):207-14, 2005.

32. Adebamowo, C.A. Spiegelman D, Berkey CS, Danby FW, Rockett HH, Colditz GA, Willett WC, Holmes MD. Milk consumption and acne in adolescent girls. Dermatol Online J; 12(4):1, 2006.

33. Adebamowo CA, Spiegelman D, Berkey CS, Danby FW, Rockett HH, Colditz GA, Willett WC, Holmes MD. Milk consumption and acne in teenaged boys. J Am Acad Dermatol. 2008 May;58(5):787-93

34. Kwon HH, Yoon JY, Hong JS, Jung JY, Park MS, Suh DH.Clinical and histological effect of a low glycaemic load diet in treatment of acne vulgaris in Korean patients: a randomized, controlled trial. Acta Derm Venereol. 2012 May;92(3):241-6

35. Bowe WP1, Joshi SS, Shalita AR. Diet and acne J Am Acad Dermatol. 2010 Jul;63(1):124-41.

36. Ismail B1, Nielsen SS. Invited review: Plasmin protease in milk: current knowledge and relevance to dairy industry. J Dairy Sci. 2010 Nov;93(11):4999-5009.

37. Rowlands MA, Gunnell D, Harris R, Vatten LJ, Holly JM, Martin RM. Circulating insulin-like growth factor peptides and prostate cancer risk: a systematic review and meta-analysis. Int J Cancer. 2009 May 15;124(10):2416-29.

38. Sugumar A, Liu YC, Xia Q, Koh YS, Matsuo K. Insulin-like growth factor (IGF)-I and IGF-binding protein 3 and the risk of premenopausal breast cancer: a meta-analysis of literature. Int J Cancer. 2004 Aug 20;111(2):293-7.

39. Qin LQ, He K, Xu JY. Milk consumption and circulating insulin-like growth factor-I level: a systematic literature review. Int J Food Sci Nutr. 2009;60 Suppl 7:330-40.

40. Rowlands MA, Gunnell D, Harris R, Vatten LJ, Holly JM, Martin RM. Circulating insulin-like growth factor peptides and prostate cancer risk: a systematic review and meta-analysis. Int J Cancer. 2009 May 15;124(10):2416-29.

41. Sugumar A, Liu YC, Xia Q, Koh YS, Matsuo K. Insulin-like growth factor (IGF)-I and IGF-binding protein 3 and the risk of premenopausal breast cancer: a meta-analysis of literature. Int J Cancer. 2004 Aug 20;111(2):293-7.

42. Genkinger JM, Hunter DJ, Spiegelman D, et al. Dairy products and ovarian cancer: a pooled analysis of 12 cohort studies. Cancer Epidemiol Biomarkers Prev. 2006 Feb;15(2):364-72

43. Larsson SC, Orsini N, Wolk A. Milk, milk products and lactose intake and ovarian cancer risk: a meta-analysis of epidemiological studies. Int J Cancer. 2006 Jan 15;118(2):431-41

44. http://www.mayo.edu/research/discoverys-edge/celiac-disease-rise

Chapter 4

Toxicities and Deficiencies - Easy Steps to Remove Environmental Toxicity and Nutritional Deficiency to Achieve the Health You Desire

Cleaning up your home may help cure a cross-section of diseases and health concerns that we have yet to find out the proper reasons as why we got them.

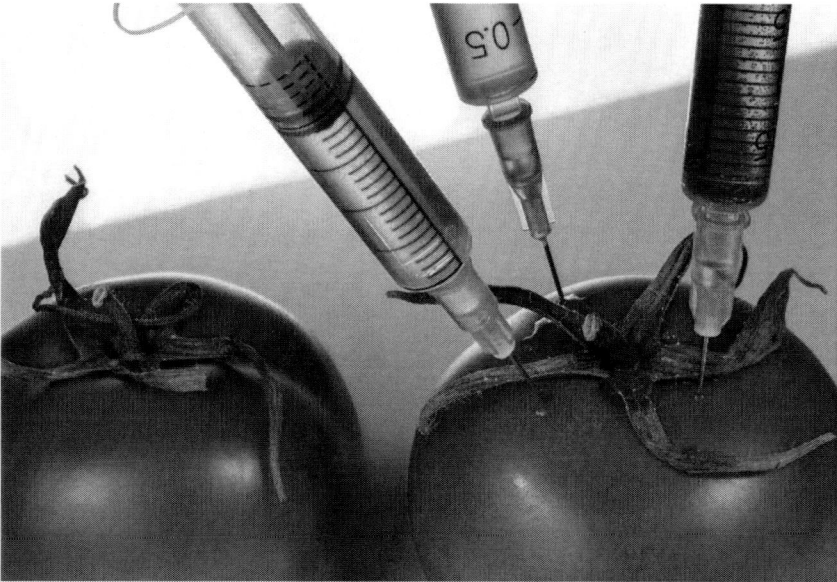

In this chapter, we look at turning toxicities and deficiencies into purity and sufficiency. We touch on environmental toxins in our home and additives in our food that may be sabotaging our health. We also address deficiencies, things that we need to be healthy in our diet that we are either not getting or not getting enough of. To be truly healthy and truly well you need be pure and sufficient.

So, what does that look like? What we have aimed to do is to give you the cliff notes on how to quickly and efficiently change your home from a toxic environment to a healthy one and how to cut back on foods containing unhealthy additives. The outcome will result in thinking more clearly, feeling more rested, having more energy during the day and being more motivated to exercise.

Additionally, for those of you who may be taking numerous nutritional supplements, you may find that with the changes you are making there may no longer be a need for extra supplements to make you feel better. We all want to feel healthy and energetic, but we often do not know how to go about achieving that. By making some simple, basic changes to your home environment and food choices, you will make a positive difference to your overall wellbeing. That is the goal and hopefully that gets you excited.

Cleaning up your home may help alleviate or eliminate all together a cross-section of diseases and health concerns that we have yet to find out the proper reasons as why we got them, but just being exposed to numerous different toxins over years and years, may result in our body breaking down because of our body's inability to continue adapting and healing from years of exposure. We recommend that you adopt these principles in your home with your family as well.

Toxins in the Home

WE THINK IN TERMS OF WELLNESS BEING DEFINED BY THE HEALTHY THINGS YOU DO MOST OF THE TIME, RATHER THAN WHAT YOU DO EVERY ONCE IN A WHILE.

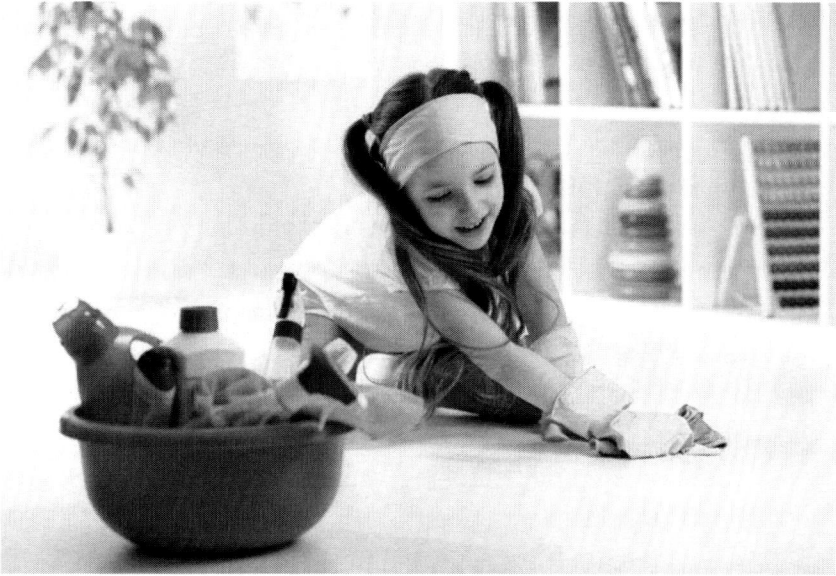

There is general consensus that air quality inside our homes is considerably more polluted than outdoor air. Recent research has shown a correlation between toxins in the home and a cross-section of health issues such as asthma, allergies, congestion and cancer. We are bombarded on a daily basis with a multitude of toxic chemicals.

The US Environmental Protection Agency (EPA) states that concentrations of volatile organic compounds (VOC) are up to ten times higher indoor than outdoors. VOCs are chemicals that are emitted indoors from a number of sources such as cigarette smoke, cleaning products, pesticides, furniture, carpets, paints, varnishes, printers, copy paper, cosmetics, air fresheners, solvents and craft materials. The EPA has published an excellent guide related to this topic that you may wish to check out www.epa.gov/iedwebo0 /pubs/hpguide.html.

It is impossible to completely eliminate exposure to all of these toxins, but we can significantly reduce our exposure by simply reducing, and whenever possible, eliminating the use of products containing toxic chemicals. Cleaning up our home may help to prevent or even cure a cross-section of diseases and health concerns for which we have yet to determine the source. Using products with toxic additives once or twice may not make much impact, however, after years of exposure particularly to numerous toxic products, our body will likely start to break down.

We think in terms of wellness being defined by the healthy things you do most of the time. It's not just the every once in a while thing. Eating an apple once or twice a month is not going to produce wellness for you, but making fresh fruits and vegetables a part of your daily diet will make a positive impact on your overall health. Likewise, if you smoke a cigar once or twice a year it's probably not going to hurt you, but smoking one every single day may be detrimental to your overall health. Our bodies will only be able to adapt so long before things start falling apart. The resulting health issues often remain undiagnosed or are misdiagnosed.

It is beyond the scope of this book to discuss the numerous environmental hazards in our home, however, we will touch on some of the most common categories of concerns. We encourage you to do further reading related to this topic. There are some excellent website resources such as the Environmental Working Group (www.ewg.org), the Environmental Protection Agency (http://householdproducts.nlm.nih.gov/) and the David Suzuki Foundation (http://www.davidsuzuki.org) websites.

Wilting Plants

Here's a neat analogy that we have used for quite a while now. We called it the Wilting Plants analogy. This comparison came from Dr. James Chestnut. Suppose you have a wilting plant in your home. The first thing you would think about is that it needs more water. So, you provide more water, but after a few days you notice that it was still dying. Would you then conclude that water was bad for the plant? Obviously not, because we know that water is essential for a plant.

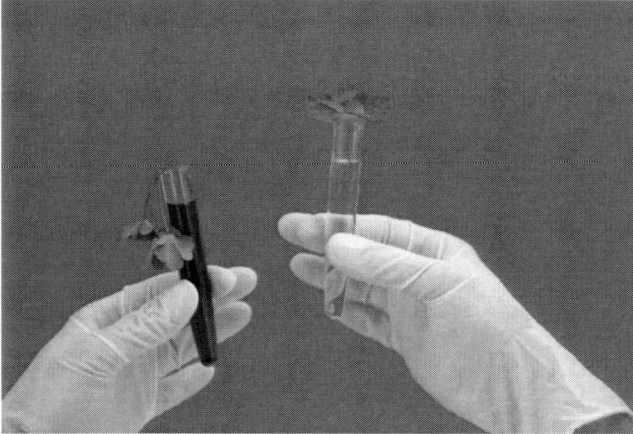

Yet it is still wilting. You then figure out that plants also need sunshine, so you put the plant in a bright spot so that it gets plenty of sun, but you notice that it is still wilting. Would you then think that sunshine is bad for the plant as well? Obviously not because we know that plants need sunshine.

So, you now have to look deeper into the situation. The plant is getting sunshine and plenty of water, so what remains to be examined is the soil the plant is in. There could be a number of problems with the soil. It could be depleted of nutrients or it could contain toxic substances. Changing the soil may make all the difference in reviving the plant back to health.

Similarly, our health could be deteriorating for a number of reasons, such as inadequate nutrition or lack of exercise. However, it could be that a toxic home environment could be "the" or "a" contributing factor in our deteriorating health. So, the next step is to clean up the toxins from our home and food to determine what difference that makes to our overall well-being.

Many of us grew up in households with medicine cabinets full of pills and exposure to pharmaceutical drug commercials on TV thinking that there is a pill for every ill.

So, if you are trying to approach health and wellness from that viewpoint, you may end up being disappointed. For example, if you have frequent headaches or migraines, you may try drinking more water because you think dehydration could be causing your headaches. But when drinking more water doesn't prevent the headaches or provide relief, it would be faulty to conclude that drinking enough water is not helpful to you. It does not mean that drinking water is a bad thing; it just was not the cure for your headache.

This situation is similar to the wilting plant. More water did not alleviate the headaches or revive the wilting plant. However, it was necessary to examine a number of possible factors, including a possibly toxic environment in order to determine the root cause of the problem. The key point here is that seldom is there a simplistic simple fix to improve our overall wellness. To say this one thing is not good for this plant because it is wilting or focusing on this one thing whether it be drinking more water or popping a pill for curing a migraine is not the answer to improved wellness. Unfortunately, we have been somewhat brainwashed to think about health and wellness in terms of quick fixes.

Removing common household toxins such as plastics, toxin-laden cosmetics, personal care products, household cleaners and aerosols may initially be a time-consuming task, but in terms of improving overall wellness, the extra effort and expense will be worth it.

CONSIDERING THAT EXPOSURE TO TOXINS IS VIRTUALLY IMPOSSIBLE TO AVOID, WHAT CAN WE DO TO STAY HEALTHY?

Indoor Toxins

BPA in Plastics

Bisphenol A (BPA) is an endocrine disrupting chemical used in the process of making plastics and resins. The message here is that BPA is a big deal because it is in a lot of the plastics as well as in in a multitude of consumer products such as plastic storage containers, baby bottles, water bottles, coffee makers, electric tea kettles, bottle tops, dental sealants and composites, as well as in epoxy resins used to line food cans. Our endocrine system is a part of our body that produces and secretes hormones, so if you are ingesting something that disrupts that system, there may be adverse health consequences that would come with that. BPA appears to stimulate the body in the same way as estrogen. This is particularly problematic as we are now also bombarded with environmental estrogens in our drinking water and in our food.

Considering that exposure to toxins is all around us and consequently virtually impossible to avoid all together, what can we do to stay healthy? What would be some alternatives to plastics and resins? Change to a wooden cutting board and perhaps cast iron, ceramic or stainless steel pots and pans. You will want to avoid Teflon and Teflon coated cookware for similar reasons because this also tends to disrupt hormonal systems in the body.

Start eliminating the plastic bowls, cups and storage containers in your home and substitute the plastic with glass, ceramic or stainless steel. Older plastic containers are particularly concerning because of the degradation of the plastic with years of wear and tear. Kids in schools are not allowed to bring glass, so an alternative could be stainless steel which may leach some metals, however this would not be nearly as toxic as the leaching from plastic. If you find it necessary or more convenient to continue to use plastic products, you can reduce exposure to BPAs by not placing hot foods in the plastic containers or exposing them to heat of any kind as the plastic may break down and leach BPA into your food. If you are purchasing plastic products check to make sure they are BPA free and not labelled with recycle codes 3 and 7 which may contain BPA.

Before the scare with BPA when I was still in school, I remember my public health professor talking about concerns with plastics. She said a good rule of thumb is if you can smell the plastic you're probably drinking it. When you take a plastic water bottle in your car and it gets hot and even after you let it cool down a lot of that plastic would likely have leached into the water. So, when you pop the cap and smell plastic, it's likely you're drinking a bit of that plastic. Again, as we mentioned before, if that happens once or twice in your life it's probably not going to be a health risk for you but if it is every single day or several times a week, year after year then that's a lot of exposure to toxicity in your life.

Replacing many questionable products does not have to be costly. It could be as simple as instead of drinking out of a plastic flip top water bottle, find one that's glass or one that's stainless steel with a flip top. It's a pretty simple thing to replace. As far as replacing cookware, plastic containers and appliances that can be done over a period of time as some of these can be costly, but they will last a long time and they are something worth saving for as it will be a good investment for your health.

Health concerns have also been noted with plastic food wrapping. Store left over food in glass containers rather than wrapping them in plastic cling wrap because of the increased potential of tiny amounts of chemicals migrating into the food particularly when used to cover fatty foods such as meat, cheese or butter. Never heat food wrapped in plastic as the risk of chemicals leaching into food is increased with heat. When lining cooking pans with parchment paper, use only unbleached parchment paper because the bleached parchment can leach dioxin, a toxic chemical and potential carcinogen. Finally, avoid canned goods and opt for fresh produce whenever possible.

With the increased public awareness and related media coverage of the harmful effects of BPA in plastics and resins, many manufacturers have responded to consumer demands to remove BPA from their products. In 2008 when Canada banned BPA from all baby bottles, the USA did not follow suit, however, consumer boycotts resulted in large retailers such as Wal-Mart to pull their BPA containing plastic baby bottles from their shelves. In 2010, Tupperware announced its products are now 100% BPA free. In 2012 Campbell's Soup announced it would begin to phase out BPAs from the lining of its cans. By 2014 products labeled "BPA-free" were commonplace. Many manufactures have now replaced BPA with bisphenol S (BPS). But how safe is this newly selected alternative? Is it equally as bad? Manufactures claim it's quite safe, but they made the same claim for BPA. Some recent research suggests that the alternatives are equally concerning. A May 2014 article by researchers, George Bittner, Chun Yang and Mathew Stoner in *Environmental Health* noted that "many BPA-free PC replacement products still leached chemicals" and that they were less biodegradable. Consequently, they would remain in your body and in the environment for extended periods of time. (http://www.ehjournal.net/content/13/1/41).

For more information related to this topic, we recommend reading *Slow Death by Rubber Duck* by Rick Smith and Bruce Lourie. The authors go into considerable depth on the effects of chemicals in Teflon and BPA and how they affect your body.

Household Cleaning Products

POTENTIALLY DANGEROUS TOXINS NOT ONLY SEEP INTO OUR BODIES BUT INTO OUR SOIL AND WATER SYSTEMS AS WELL

Many of the cleaning products we use in our home contain toxic chemicals that penetrate our skin or that we breathe into our bodies. A great resource is the Environmental Working Group (www.ewg.org). They have several handouts that you can download and print out. One is called the 'Environmental Working Group's Cleaner's Database Hall of Shame' and it is a fairly quick visual read. The data base lists different types of cleaning products that masquerade as natural or green but are not and quite the contrary, as they produce a lot of fumes, are quite toxic and simply should not be in your home at all. The David Suzuki Foundation is another recommended site that provides a useful reference list of toxic chemicals in household cleaning products (http://www.davidsuzuki.org/issues/health/science/toxics/the-dirt-on-toxic-chemicals-in-household-cleaning-products/).

Some of our common household cleaners contain hazardous toxic chemicals. We will touch on a few of these. The purpose of highlighting some of the toxins in products you may use on a regular basis is to encourage you to read the labels and to do your own research. The toxin 2-Butoxyethanol (2-BE), which has been shown to cause blood disorders, can be found in products such as glass, carpet and oven cleaners and in concentrations as high as 22 per cent in laundry stain removers.

Ammonia, found in many household cleaners, is a skin and lung irritant, but more concerning is that ammonia is often mixed with product containing chlorine bleach resulting in the formation of a highly poisonous gas. Most cleaning products contain unnecessary coal tar dyes which have been linked to cancer and nervous system disorders. Phthalates associated with endocrine disruption and reduced sperm count, benzene, formaldehyde and a number of volatile organic compounds (VOCs) linked with cancer are found in air fresheners, laundry detergents, softeners and many household cleaning products.

Anti-bacterial agents such as triclosan and quaternary ammonium compounds (quats) found in bathroom cleaners, fabric softeners, cosmetics and other household cleaning products have been linked to antibiotic resistant bacteria. Silica powder found in abrasive powder cleaners is hazardous if inhaled. Sodium dichloroisocyanurate dihydrate is linked to kidney damage. Caustic soda or lye, a respiratory and skin irritant. Sodium lauryl sulfate (SLS), another skin irritant and potential carcinogen, are found in toilet bowel and oven cleaners and disinfectants. Trisodium nitrilotriacetate, linked to cancer, is found in bathroom cleaners. These potentially dangerous toxins not only seep into our bodies but into our soil and water systems as well.

Removing household products containing potentially harmful toxins can be done over a period of time. As you finish off the concerning products replace them with safer alternatives. We use some Norwex products in our home. They have cleaning towels, rags and mops that have silver embedded into the material which is a natural antimicrobial and it is great because you do not have to use any cleaning solutions at all. It is basically just water and the rag or water and a mop and it basically has the same effect as if you were to use cleaning products containing chemicals. For about $20.00 or $30.00 you can replace all of your dishrags and mop. We use ours every single day and they don't seem to wear out. Check the websites and the lists of ingredients (http://norwex.biz/). There are several alternatives in the market place.

Cosmetics and Body Products

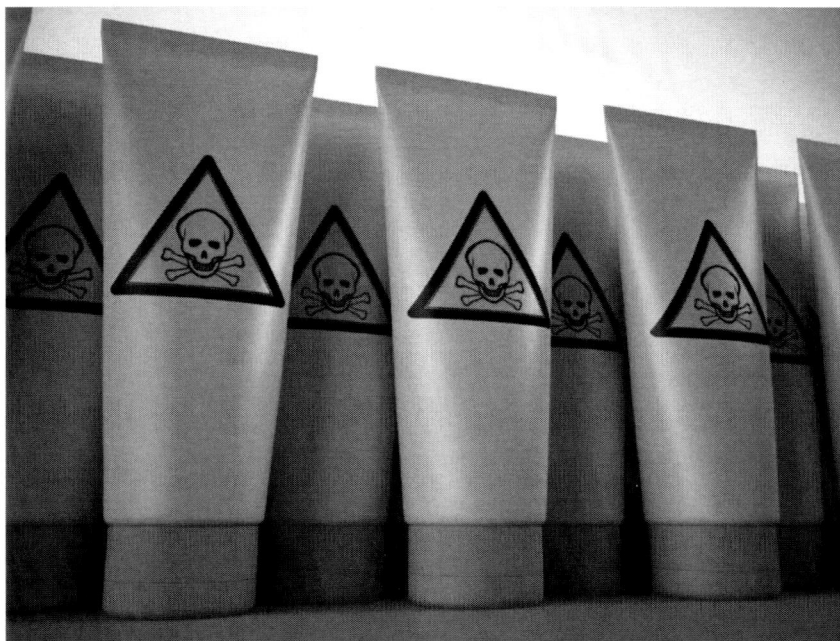

Several websites provide convenient reference lists of toxic chemicals to avoid when purchasing cosmetics or body products. The David Suzuki Foundation website has a list of products to avoid, called the Dirty Dozen. They are: BHA & BHT, Coal tar dyes,Cyclomethicone & siloxanes, DEA, MEA & TEA, Dibutyl phthalate, Formaldehyde. Parabens, Parfum (a.k.a fragrance), PEG compounds, Petrolatum, SLES & SLS and Triclosan (http://www.davidsuzuki.org/issues/health/science/toxics/dirty-dozen-cosmetic-chemicals/).

These are the primary chemicals that we need to avoid when it comes to cosmetics, shampoos, and bath products. You will even find three of the listed concerning toxins in toothpaste, sodium lauryl sulfate (SLS), sodium laureth sulfate (SLES) and triclosan, Chronic exposure to these chemicals over time is the problem.

I think a good rule of thumb is to try and go as close back to nature as you can. If you read the ingredients and there are thirty-five ingredients and they include toxic chemicals, it is probably not something you want to put on your body. There are healthier alternatives. The shampoo and body wash that we use is a relatively inexpensive organic shea butter based product consisting of three main ingredients, a coconut oil surfactant, organic lavender and lavender essential oil. Our entire family uses it. It works well and has a pleasant lavender essential oil scent.

If you check the websites and do some comparison shopping, you can find good quality toxin-free products for reasonable prices. Often these products are more concentrated so you will not have to use nearly as much. They are not going to foam up the same way because they don't have the chemical foaming agents added, but you will get used to that fairly quickly. There are numerous websites that have good resources. We both use the Green Polka Dot Box (http://www.greenpolkadotbox.com/). They have a large selection of products. If you are in a community that does not have a natural grocery you may consider getting these products online.

With make-up and skincare products, read the ingredient lists and if it states that it is natural or mineral based, but the ingredients show that there are numerous chemicals, it is probably not okay, but on the other hand, if there are just three or four different minerals then, of course, that is a much better option.

Sunscreens and bug repellents that many of us use especially during the summer months can be concerning. Many sunscreens contain toxic chemicals that block the sun and stimulate cells in the skin predisposing it to skin cancer, which is ironic because the whole point of sunscreen is to protect you from the UV rays but then when it is carcinogenic and stimulates cancer growth in the skin, what is the point in that. There are a number of basic sunscreens on the market such as the zinc-based sunscreens which have been around for a long time but are not popular because they are white and reflect the light.

Dr. Mercola's Tree Oil zinc oxide-based sunscreen is another consideration (products.mercola.com/sunscreen). It works well and also has water repellent properties. There are a number of other safe sunscreens available on-line and in stores. Of course, we do need some sun rays because that is what produces Vitamin D and higher Vitamin D levels lower the risk of skin cancer. Moderation is the key.

Insect Repellants and Pesticides

There are still some bug repellents with DEET on the market. Stay away from these products. They work well to keep mosquitoes away but DEET is a known carcinogen, so if you are thinking of dousing your children with these bug repellants to prevent a few mosquito bites, it is a poor trade off given the risk of cancer and other problems arising from that.

There are a number of healthy options such as Burt's Bees which includes citronella oil and pine tree oil. It does not work as well as the DEET but it is none-the-less a good option. It smells great and you don't feel like you need to go home and wash it off right away. With pesticides and herbicides there are some alternatives. For example, chrysanthemum extracts can be used to spray hornet and wasp nests. It is not harmful to humans but it is destructive to the nervous system of the wasps. Again, check the ingredients on the labels. There are a lot of things on the market that masquerade as natural, but just because it says natural on the label it does not necessarily mean it is.

EMF Pollution

Another concern is EMF pollution in the home. EMF stands for Electromagnetic Frequencies. It is definitely a topic many people do not think about much, however, there is a lot of new research showing the problems with these frequencies. One of the biggest exposures is the waterbed heater. If you sleep on a waterbed, the electric heater that you are laying on emits a lot of EMF.

The new flat screen televisions create huge electromagnetic exposure, so it is wise not to sit too close. If you have your cell phone in your pocket, sit in front of the computer all day long, sit in front of your TV in the evening, lay on a heated waterbed at night surrounded by electronics around you, routers, phones, et cetera, then all these different things will be emitting EMF. Turning the power off some of these devices when not in use plus trying to minimize your exposure to them can help. There are a number of products on the market that can help to reduce EMF emissions. A small disk-shaped stick on device that can be attached to your cell phone, exposure reducing floor mats to place around your computer and Q-Link pendants and bracelets are just some examples of available products.

Paints and Varnishes

Paints and varnishes can be quite toxic to the nervous system. There are some water based acrylic clear coat varathanes on the market that have no odor at all and they are about the same price. There are also other safer paints and varathanes that will cost a little bit more, but then how often do you paint your home or a room so spending a little bit more to avoid toxic chemical exposures is worth a few extra dollars.

Synthetic Furniture and Carpeting

Synthetic furniture and carpets emit toxic chemicals into the air. Particularly concerning are new carpets. Cleaning the carpets adds to the problem as many carpet cleaning products can contain numerous dangerous toxic ingredients such as formaldehyde, perchlorethylene and 2-butoxy ethanol.

Household Appliances

Household appliances such as gas stoves, space heaters, furnaces and fireplaces release toxins such as nitrogen dioxide, carbon monoxide and methane into the air.

Aerosols

"Our understanding of the literature is that there is no such thing as safe use of most volatile solvents, aerosols or other street inhalants: psychoactive effects may be inseparable from nerve and organ damage." (www.Erowid.org)

Aerosols are particularly concerning. Aerosols ranging from shaving creams to cleaning products can contain formaldehyde and phenol and carcinogens such as benzene and xylene. Research has shown that even a few seconds of exposure to these chemicals can result in these toxins penetrating organs in our body.

Chemicals and Preservatives in Our Food

Over 10,000 chemicals are permitted in our food. (www.ewg.org)

Another huge category are chemicals and preservatives in our everyday foods. The Environmental Working Group (EWG) notes that over 10,000 chemicals are permitted in our food. Some of these additives are chemicals linked to serious health concerns such as endocrine disruption, allergies, hyperactivity in children, nerve disorders and cancer. To help consumers decide which foods should be avoided, the EWG has published an excellent resource, the *Dirty Dozen Guide to Food Additives*, a list of the most concerning additives to avoid (www.ewg.org/research/ewg-s-dirty-dozen-guide-food-additives**).** There are a number of other good website resources that address this topic. An example is: http://articles.mercola.com/sites/articles/archive/2014/11/26/12 -worst-food-additives.aspx.

With such an overwhelming number of additives in our food what can we do as consumers to find healthy options? We recommend you check out the list of product ingredients, look for products with the fewest number of ingredients and avoid all foods with additives that are linked to health concerns. Select fresh, non-processed or minimally processed foods and avoid packaged or boxed foods and cured meats whenever possible. If there are 35 ingredients on the label, you probably should not be eating it. Unfortunately, it is the children who are consuming most of the processed foods with artificial food colorings and other potentially harmful additives.

Aim to eat basic, natural, locally-grown and organic food whenever possible. For example, when you choose free range natural chicken you are just eating chicken rather than chicken with phosphates, hormones and added fillers. Similarly, when choosing free range organic eggs, you are assured of a safer, more nutritious option. Eat a banana instead of a box of crackers _ just simple things. The key message here is to aim to get back to what are natural, basic foods.

Once again, we don't want to try and be fanatical about this. If you consume processed foods now and then it is probably not going to be a big deal. Your body will adapt to it, but if you eat these processed foods on a regular basis there is a risk of health problems developing. Start with one or two things at a time. Maybe you really like your diet soda but you are aware that artificial sweeteners in soda have been implicated with health problems so perhaps that's the place you should start. Replace it with green tea, water or something else and once you tackle that then go on to the next thing.

There is no right or wrong way to go about it. We will provide you with some alternatives, things that you can substitute, but you can also come up with your own plan. Decide what are the big things in your life that you would like to change. Do you want to drink clean water or eat more natural or organic pesticide free foods? The approach you take to cleaning up your body will depend on where you are currently at. The Environmental Working Group has a great list for shopping, 'A Shopper's Guide to Produce' that lists which fruits and vegetables have the most exposure to pesticides and those which have the least exposure (http://www.ewg.org/foodnews/). You may be surprised to learn that apples, strawberries, grapes and celery are on top of the list for pesticide exposure, while avocado, sweet corn, pineapples and cabbage have the least. Refer to the guide when deciding what foods you should buy organic. With many foods, it is safer and more nutritious to eat organic. Of course, when you're thinking about organic you are also thinking about non-genetically modified foods, but that goes into a whole other discussion, so just take a step at a time.

Nutritional Sufficiency

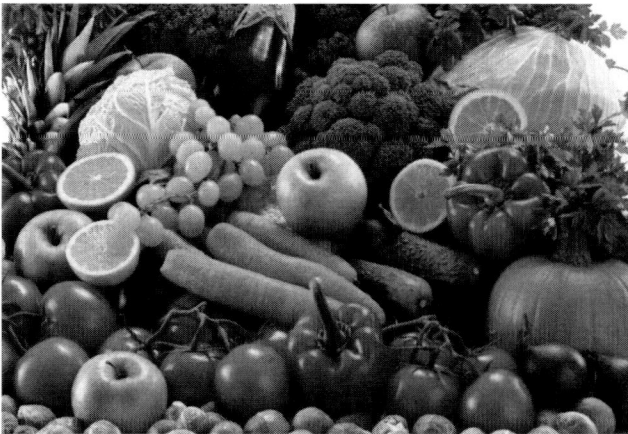

What is meant by Nutritional Sufficiency? What is the idea behind sufficiency? We do not like to promote large quantities of supplements. So If you are eating a healthy diet, what are some things you may still be deficient in? We want to create that sufficiency. To do that there are only a few things that need to be supplemented in one's diet unless you are treating a specific condition.

Vitamin D3

One of the vitamins that generally needs supplementation is vitamin D3. It is interesting that there is no adequate dietary source for vitamin D. It is as if we were intended to get it from the sun, but obviously most of us work indoors now and use sunscreens when we are outdoors, consequently we are not getting enough sunshine to produce the vitamin D we need. Ideally, we should be getting our D levels measured to see where we are at. What amounts of Vitamin D we should be taking is still up for debate. The Mayo Clinic recommends a daily dosage of 600 IUs. for healthy individuals, but also notes that higher dosages are used to treat various health conditions (http://www.mayoclinic.org/drugs-supplements/vitam in-d/dosing/HRB-20060400).

A lot of people are scared of overdosing on vitamin D, but for adults not suffering from Vitamin D sensitivity, taking daily doses of up to 10,000 or 20,000 IUs has not shown to produce a toxic effect. Toxicity has been shown in some cases in daily dosages over 50,000 IUs. Higher doses have been administered for brief periods of time under medical supervision to treat certain medical conditions. In any case, since Vitamin D can have side effects for some individuals with vitamin D sensitivity or when taken in very high doses, it is always prudent to check with a health professional if you have questions or concerns.

On the flip side of the coin, there is considerable current research related to the potential health risks that may result from not having enough vitamin D, ranging from osteoporosis, to depression, to fertility issues and even to increased cancer risks. So, if anything, perhaps we are being overly cautious with vitamin D. It is a fat-soluble vitamin that tends to be stored in the liver. In the past, there was a concern about fat-soluble vitamins and toxins, but perhaps we erred too far on the side of avoiding vitamin D. Getting vitamin D solely from our food and the sun has proven to be inadequate. If possible, we recommend a vitamin D blood test to find a baseline score of where you are at and then based on the results decide on the best dosage. You can ask your family doctor to refer you for testing or try to find a reasonably priced laboratory on your own. Also, check to see if there are health fairs in your area doing blood testing.

Whole Food Nutritional Supplements

When taking vitamins, we recommend you take whole food supplements because artificial or synthetic vitamins are missing a lot of co-factors that are necessary to get proper utilization of those nutrients. If you think you are missing certain things in your diet, whole food multivitamins can be a good insurance policy to fill in the gaps and most of these whole food multivitamins are going to be natural organic minerals. As well, the whole food products are broken down and contain different enzymes like papaya, pineapple, a little bit of probiotic, natural minerals, natural vitamin D and some D3, natural vitamin A, natural vitamin E. Most of your whole food vitamins are going to have the naturally occurring vitamins as their source.

Fish Oil

We have heard a lot about Omega 3 fats and fish oil. The concern here is that we are not getting enough fats in our diet anymore. Part of the problem is the anti-fat obsession we have had over the last twenty years or so and that is creating a deficiency in those essential fatty acids. Omega 3 fats get incorporated in every cell of the body. They make up our brain, nervous system, our skin, bones, hair. In fact, everything in our body utilizes Omega 3 fats, so it's essential that we get these good fats for optimal health.

Research has shown that even someone who has not had a great diet and has been eating a lot of unhealthy trans fats which can get incorporated in the cell membrane, in the course of three to six months of substituting and replacing those bad fats with good fats these cell membranes will replace the unhealthy fats with healthy fats. So if you are looking at someone who is having some bouts of depression and issues with the neurotransmission activity in the brain, all of that may be caused by a deficiency of good healthy fats. The nerve cells just aren't firing off right, so in the course of a few months if you start replacing the bad fats with good fats the brain will start to work right again. We have seen that with kids with learning disabilities.

We do not want to suggest that you make fish oil a treatment for disease but the neat thing is that your body is always repairing and replacing cells so if you start to put the good stuff into your body it will incorporate those into the cells.

Probiotics

Probiotics are the good bacteria essential for proper body functioning. They live in our gut and 80% of our immune function comes from gut health. Probiotics help with digestion and the production of certain vitamins and other essential processes that contribute to our immune system.

It is worth mentioning that we are currently born into a rather sterile world. The hospitals are sterilized, our fruits and vegetables are irradiated to kill any possible E.coli or other organisms, a lot of our meat and other products are also sterile, so we are not getting that natural flora that we need. Again, in a perfect world we would be getting healthy bacteria naturally in our food, but in our imperfect world we are simply not consuming sufficient amounts of beneficial bacteria. If your diet is not optimal and you are consuming foods with a lot of preservatives and artificial colorings that may kill off the good bacteria, supplementing with probiotics would be wise.

Hydration

There are a whole host of health issues that come with chronic dehydration, such as headaches or migraines. Physiologically our bodies require a certain amount of water for chemical processes to happen naturally in the body, so if you are chronically dehydrated those processes are just not going to function properly. Additionally, ensure that you are drinking clean water. In certain situations, it is best to drink properly filtered water as some tap water can contain toxins such as aluminum, arsenic, pesticides, chlorinated hydrocarbons, chlorine, and fluoride which may affect IQ, bones and tissue calcification.

There are a number of reasons as to why some people are dehydrated. The amount of water we should drink will depend on a number of factors such as our daily routines. A construction worker working outside during hot weather will require more water than someone working indoors at a desk job. The outside worker will obviously be perspiring a lot more. Is there a rule-of-thumb to go by here? One rule-of-thumb would be drinking half your body weight in ounces. This is a good way to make sure you are not deficient as far as hydration goes. It is a great place to start. If you are eating large amounts of raw vegetables and things with a high water content you probably do not need to drink that much water, however, a lot will depend on what you are doing with the rest of your diet. A good way to think about it is that if you wait until you are thirsty then you are already dehydrated.

The wilting plant comes to mind. If a plant is wilting and you douse it with water, it will not be instantly hydrated. The root of the plant must absorb the moisture and that again is not instant. So, if you feel thirsty and you drink a glass of water you are not hydrating, rather, that water is just sitting in your stomach for a period of time and eventually will go into your bloodstream and the cells. Think about a dried out sponge that is sitting on your window ledge. If you put it under the faucet initially it is just going to bead off that water: it needs to take some time to absorb that water.

Action Plan

These are things you will want to incorporate and continue on as you pursue your health and wellness. Some baby steps for the month would be to start to eliminate some of these toxins in your home and environment. Again, create your own action plan for how that may look. We will have a downloadable action plan for you. http://thewellnesssolution.co/wp-content/uploads/2015/06/mod -4-handout-V2.pdf. Another great resource to find out if the products you use are safe is the Environmental Working Group Site, http://www.ewg.org/skindeep.

Just start with baby steps. If it is daunting absorbing all this information, that is totally fine. Simply start by focusing on one area at a time while working towards achieving your desired level of nutrition and sufficiency. Perhaps you will choose to do some research and go to a vitamin store to check out some whole foods and whole food supplements. There are a number of good websites sites we have mentioned that you can examine. With hydration, some of you may be right where you need to be and others may not even drink water as your hydration comes through foods, milk, fruit juices and soda or other places. Everyone has needs that are a bit different.

You may find too that as you start drinking water you will begin to crave water. We have patients who say that they cannot stand the taste of water. It is just one of those things that you have to become accustomed to. Once your body is getting what it wants it will start to crave those things. You can also add a little bit of lemon or lime juice to the water for flavor. Some water can be borderline acidic so a slice of lemon is a great way to alkalize the water and add a little bit of flavor. A lot of people do not realize that even though lemon is acidic, it is alkalizing the body.

We have covered a lot of material in this chapter. We encourage you to download all of the forms, handouts, action plans, action steps, three-hole punch them, put them in a binder and start to create some organization with all of this material. We definitely recommend that you come back and look at these handouts again. Continue with the exercises and dietary changes. It's all about baby steps. Do not feel like it is information overload. Just take a step at a time. Keep in mind that wellness is a continuous journey, always changing and evolving.

Chapter 5

Demystifying Medications, Supplements and Common Diseases

In this chapter we cover common medications, essential supplements and common diseases. I do not think there is anyone who would dispute the face that medications are overused and often unnecessary. What are the alternatives? What supplements, if any, should I be taking? These are just some of the questions covered in this chapter.

Problems with Medications

NO MEDICATION CAN FIX A POOR LIFESTYLE.

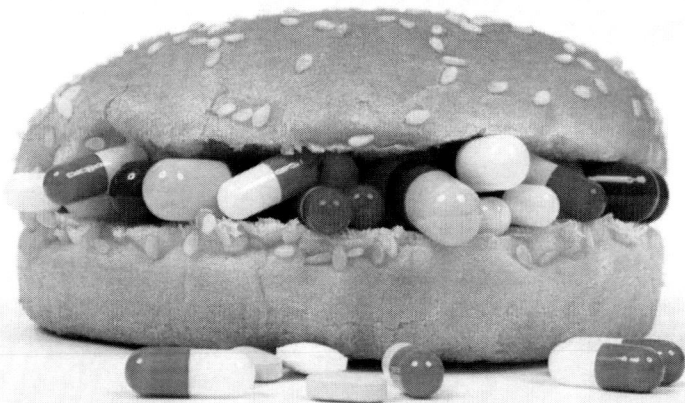

No medication can fix poor lifestyles. Nor, can medication fix nutritional deficiencies. All medication comes with inherent side effects and risks. Most, if not all medications are developed to treat symptoms of chronic disease. They can alleviate these symptoms, but they cannot produce health.

At the outset, we want to make it clear that we are not opposed to medications that could be lifesaving, such as antibiotics or insulin which may be necessary for acute life-threatening conditions. We are not talking about medications that are necessary. Obviously, in life-threatening situations, medication may be the only option, however, they are often over used and may even be harmful or dangerous. It is definitely something you have to watch.

So, what are some the problems with medications and the taking of medications? As we mentioned, there are situations when they are necessary and lifesaving, At the same time, we see how our poor lifestyles have created certain underlying conditions and diseases. It appears that many pharmaceutical companies are developing medications for these chronic lifestyle diseases, although we know no medication can cure or fix poor lifestyles. Obviously, if these medications are being developed simply to treat the symptoms of poor lifestyles, then there is no end in sight for that or for fixing the poor lifestyles that created the symptoms in the first place. In other words, in these situations there is no correcting the cause of the problem.

In 2011, doctors in the United States wrote over 4 billion prescriptions. That works out to approximately thirteen prescriptions for every man, woman and child – about one per month. Each year more than 100, 00 people die from improperly prescribed medications. (http://www.naturalnews.com/037226 _drug_prescriptions_medical_news_pills.html)

The United States Centers for Disease Control and Prevention states that there has been a steady increase of drug-induced deaths. In 2010, 38,329 people died of drug overdose. Of these, approximately sixty per cent were related to prescription drugs. By 2013, the reported drug-induced deaths had climbed to

43,982 (http://www.cdc.gov/media/releases/2013/p0220_drug_overdose_deaths.html).

The overuse of prescription drugs is particularly acute with the elderly, especially when hospitalized or in residential care (www.cdc.gov/media/releases/2011/p1123_elderly_risk.html; www.cdc.gov/nchs/pressroom/04news/elderly.htm).

In the industrialized world, we in the United States hold the bragging rights for consuming the bulk of the medications– much more than any other industrialized nation. Obviously, there is a serious problem with the current system.

It is not possible for medications to produce health. If we want to create health in our lives, medications cannot do that. Medications are often prescribed for life because people are not changing the aspects in their lifestyles that may have caused the disease process in the first place. As we have mentioned, medication on its own will never fix problems caused by poor lifestyle choices.

However, we stress again that medication is necessary in a number of situations. For example, medication may be necessary for Type 2 diabetics to control their blood sugar levels, but at the same time it is not going to fix the problem which has been brought on by poor lifestyle choices. To change that, the individuals will need to modify their lifestyle which may include eating better, exercising more and perhaps losing weight. Once these lifestyle modifications have been made, Type 2 diabetics may be able to reduce their medication or come off their medication completely. However, it is important to clarify that Type 1 diabetes, which at present has no known cause, is not the result of poor lifestyle choices. With Type 1 diabetes, insulin currently is necessary to control blood sugar levels, but at the same time healthy lifestyle choices are essential to maintain optimum health.

Another big problem with medications is that taking medications for long periods of time, especially different types of medications, can result in greater nutritional deficiencies. Statin drugs, for example, are drugs taken when your cholesterol is high.

These statin drugs often block an enzyme in your liver called CO Enzyme Q10 which is important for muscle and cardiac functions in the body. These statin drugs block the production of that particular nutrient and over time can create other health effects as well. In particular it can trigger migraines and cause problems with muscle function and circulatory issues.

The longer you take these statin drugs, the greater the risk will be that you will develop nutritional deficiencies because of the interaction of that drug in your body. If the expectation is for you to continue taking this drug over a long-term period, it is important to carefully weigh your options.

Drugs, such as estrogens and hormone replacement therapies may deplete vitamin B and magnesium, while antibiotic are known to deplete the beneficial bacteria in the gut. If that is not replaced quickly then virulent bacteria may develop. Other medications such as antidepressants which are often prescribed long term can deplete melatonin and throw off the thyroid. Another group of drugs prescribed long term, often for life, are blood pressure medications. These are situations where we can start to see interactions and deficiencies develop.

SOME DRUGS CAN PERPETUATE OR EVEN EXHASPERATE THE PROBLEM YOU ARE TRYING TO ALLEVIATE.

Some drugs can perpetuate the problem you are trying to alleviate or eliminate. Some medications prescribed for sleep for example, might decrease melatonin levels which are necessary for proper sleep functioning. Consequently, the prescribed sleep medication exasperates the problem which in turn perpetuates the need for the medication. Similarly, long term use of migraine and headache medication over time will trigger a migraine. Antidepressants have also been linked to exacerbating the problem they are prescribed to resolve. There have been numerous studies in the past few years that show that chronic use of antidepressants will over time cause depression and possible thoughts of suicide. It is important to keep in mind that the use of these drugs can create the opposite effect.

At the end of this chapter we provide links to hand outs on this topic. You may want to print out this supplementary information and take it to your family doctor to discuss lifestyle modifications and possible reductions or changes to your current medications.

Common Medications

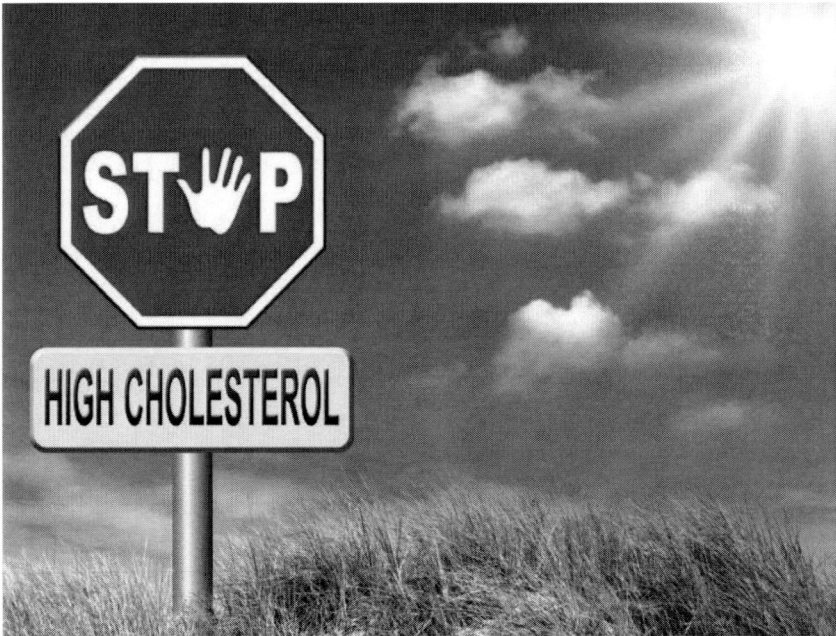

In this chapter, we touch on some of the most prescribed common medications. We are not going to dig too deep into each medication, but just take the bird's eye view of each. As previously mentioned, most of these medications are designed to treat the symptoms of poor lifestyle. Part of the problem with these medications, when you look at it from a pharmaceutical stand point, is that it seems these companies are looking to having you, their patients, on these medications for a lifetime.

When you are on these medications for longer periods of time, the concern is that you can become dependent on these drugs. Your body stops doing what it is supposed to be doing naturally because it no longer needs to be doing these functions on its own. As a result, your body creates less of a need to work towards self-healing which makes your body rely on those extra medications to help support the body functions. When you think about a function in the body that is no longer working properly, it creates a symptom which can include pain or inflammation. We then treat the symptom with medication. Consequently, at no point in the process are we fixing the underlying problem.

Cholesterol Medication

Prescriptions for cholesterol medications have shown a steady increase over the past decade. Cholesterol medications are the second most prescribed medication in the United States. (http://www.medscape.com/viewarticle/825053). Side effects can include stomach & digestive issues, muscle cramps, soreness, pain and weakness. High cholesterol in and of itself is not a problem. There are a lot of different factors that go into heart disease. Inflammation is one of these.

So, if you just look at one particular thing and think you need to medicate this particular problem, you are missing the big picture. High cholesterol, poor lifestyle, high stress, and high inflammation - those are the type of things that lead to cardiovascular disease. If the body is under excessive stress from physical biochemical, emotional or other causes, your body will produce more cholesterol as an adaptive response to deal with this stress. Consequently, if you have a medication that artificially lowers cholesterol, your body is going to try harder to make more cholesterol, but it is not going to fix the problem. Conversely, it will create other problems that you are going to have to deal with while ignoring the underlying issue which is excessive stress that has not been dealt with.

The human body is an amazingly designed piece of machinery that does not make mistakes. It is going to do what it needs to do to adapt to the environment. So, when you see high cholesterol, instead of thinking you need to go on medication, you should ask why the cholesterol is so high in the first place. Having high cholesterol for a short period of time is not going to kill you. You are not going to get a heart attack from that. Obviously, with stress hormones high, with inflammation high, with cholesterol high eroding the arteries over time, these are obvious concerns that must be addressed. From a health care standpoint, we need to look at why this is happening.

Narcotic Analgesics

PAIN IS AN ADAPTIVE RESPONSE TO SOMETHING ELSE GOING ON IN YOUR BODY. MASKING PAIN IS NOT GOING TO SOLVE THE PROBLEM.

Narcotic analgesics are your common opiate-based pain relievers available only by prescription. These are frequently prescribed for pain and pose dangers of addiction intoxication and overdose risks. Approx. 27,500 people died from unintentional drug overdose in 2007 driven to a large extent by prescription opiate overdose. Fortunately, we are seeing fewer and fewer of these prescribed because the DEA has cracked down on these medications especially from a chronic pain stand point, but even so there are approximately 30,000 deaths per year from the use of these medications from overdosing.

Many individuals taking these medications are driving vehicles and even operating machinery. Research has shown that the longer you are on these medications the greater the probability will be that you may end up developing the underlying problem you are trying to treat with the particular medication. For example, as we stated earlier, if you are trying to treat migraines, over time the medication can start to create headaches or migraines, so it is a chronic approach to a particular problem. Not surprisingly, pharmaceutical companies put the lion's share of their dollars to these types of medications because of the projected profits.

Again, pain is just an adaptive response to something else going on, so masking this pain with medication is not going to solve the problem. It can be very beneficial and necessary at times but it should be looked at as a short term situation while trying to determine what the actual cause of the problem is.

Anti-depressants

Anti-depressants are among the top prescribed medications in the United States. Concerns related to over-use of antidepressant and antipsychotic drugs for seniors in nursing homes and hospitals has recently been highlighted. A recent study conducted in British Columbia, Canada noted that 34% of seniors in residential care are on prescription antipsychotic drugs, although only 4% have been diagnosed with a mental disorder (as reported April 10, 2015, Vancouver Sun Newspaper, BC Canada). These brain-altering drugs can have serious side-effects ranging from insomnia, agitation and aggressive or violent behavior to thoughts of suicide. There are many ways to alleviate depression naturally. These include EFT (Emotional freedom technique), exercise, sunshine, omega 3 fats, probiotics, and improving general nutrition. (http://articles.mercola.com/sites/articles/archive/2011/03/07/r eversing-depression-without-antidepressants.aspx)

Beta Blocker

Beta blockers are prescribed for high blood pressure, as well as glaucoma, hyperthyroidism and migraines. There were more than 195 million prescriptions in the United States in 2010. Side effects include headaches, cold hands, constipation, diarrhea, dizziness, sleep problems, shortness of breath, depression and rapid heartbeat. Beta blockers can be particularly dangerous for asthmatics because they can trigger asthma attacks and for diabetics because they can block readings for low blood sugar levels. (http://www.mayoclinic.org/diseases-conditions/)

ACE Inhibitors and Angiotensin

ACE inhibitors and Angiotensin are also prescribed for high blood pressure as well as for scleroderma and migraines. In 2010 pharmacies dispensed more than 168.7 million prescriptions for ACE inhibitors. There are numerous possible side effects - anxiety, dizziness, headaches, fatigue, anemia, depression, swelling of legs or ankles, bleeding gums, to poor healing and even to thoughts of suicide. (http://www.mayoclinic.org/diseases-conditions/)

Many natural ways that can reduce blood pressure exist. These include a healthy diet which is discussed at length throughout The Wellness Solution. In particular, decreasing fructose, grains, caffeine and sugar while increasing omega 3 fats and other healthy fats, fermented foods and Vitamin D. Some other helpful suggestions can be found here. http://articles.mercola.com/sites/articles/archive/2010/10/08/discover-the-secret-to-lowering-your-blood-pressure-in-15-minutes.aspx

Thyroid Medications

Thyroid medication is the most prescribed medication in the United States with approximately 23 million prescriptions in 2014 (based on the most recent IMS Health research data in http://www.medscape.com/viewarticle/825053).

Individuals who express symptoms such as chronic fatigue, poor concentration, cold hands, hair loss, fluid retention or depression may have low thyroid. Hypothyroidism results when the thyroid gland is no longer able to create sufficient thyroid hormones to maintain a healthy body. The American Thyroid Association states that there is no cure once diagnosed and advocates a combination of a drug-based approach supplemented by a diet with iodine-rich foods such as fish and kelp (http://www.thyroid.org) problem is that there is a danger that hyperthyroidism can be misdiagnosed and thyroid hormones taken unnecessarily resulting in drugs such as levothyroxine being recommended for life.

Going on thyroid medication based on a single blood test result can be concerning. It is not unusual for blood test results to vary from one test to the other. It is important for you to take control of your own health and to explore all available options. There have been numerous instances where an individual has shown symptoms of hyperthyroidism at a particular time, but after following a healthy diet and regular exercise schedule these symptoms have dissipated. A good healthy lifestyle should also be the first step. Thyroid medication can have numerous side effects ranging from anxiety and irritability to rapid heartbeat to weight loss.

Taking synthetic thyroid medications treats the symptoms but it does not fix the underlying problem. The longer you are on thyroid medication the more you have to take the medication because your body adjusts to the need for the medication. Over time, you no longer need to make your own thyroid hormones because you are creating them artificially. We do want to stress that it is not wise to self-treat hypothyroidism. We recommend you take both blood tests and temperature tests if you suspect you may have a low thyroid because neither blood nor temperature tests on their own are always conclusive. The late Dr. Brody Barnes, a Colorado physician created a printable chart to track your temperature (http://www.thewolfeclinic.com/barnes-thyroid-temperature-test/). However, it is important to highlight that temperature tests which have been subject to controversy should not be used as conclusive evidence of a low thyroid. Always consult with an alternative health care provider familiar with treating thyroid issues if you suspect a thyroid problem. If you wish to find more information on thyroid temperature testing, there are a number of websites you can check out.

Other Medications

Other commonly prescribed medications are diuretics, hormonal contraceptives, ulcer medications, antibiotics, diabetic and respiratory medication. However, it is beyond the scope of this book to address all of these. Suffice it to say that, before taking medications, do your homework and become an informed advocate for your own health.

Supplements: What do you really need?

THE BULK OF HEALTH CARE FOCUSES ON A REACTIVE RATHER THAN A PREVENTATIVE APPROACH

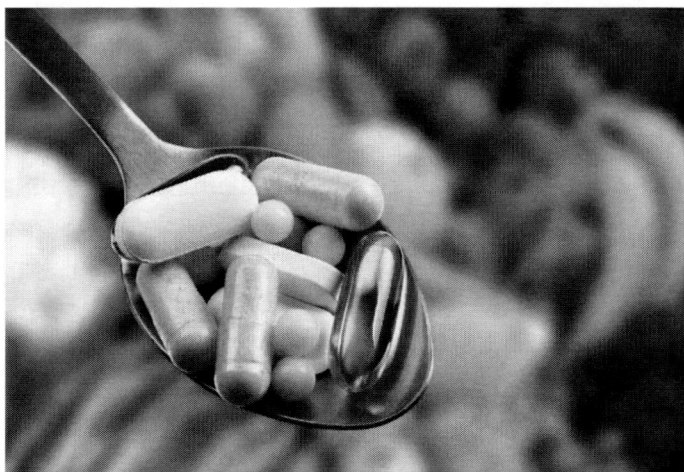

Next in this chapter, we move away from medications and address supplements. Are supplements necessary? You often hear or read that supplements are unnecessary if you follow a healthy diet. However, there is increasing concern that the average American diet does not contain sufficient amounts of nutrients to maintain optimum health. How do we know if we need additional supplementation and how much is enough? Can we trust the advertising? After all, these companies are out to make money by selling as much of their products as possible. Can we rely on our family physicians when the primary focus of their training has focused mostly on pharmaceutical treatments and only a few hours have been spent on nutritional education in medical school? Or do we follow the recommendations of high-profile physicians such as Doctors Mehmet Oz, Andrew Weil, Gifford-Jones, William Davis or David Heber? All of these physicians support the use of nutritional supplementations.

Dr. David Heber, Director of the UCLA Center for Human Nutrition and Chief of the Division of Clinical Nutrition in the Department of Medicine at the University of California, Los Angeles (http://ccim.med.ucla.edu/) claims that natural supplements have the potential to "significantly lower their risk of a multitude of serious diseases" (conference for the Council on Responsible Nutrition, March 31, 1998). It is easy to feel confused with so many mixed messages.

The bulk of health care entails a reactive approach that focuses on treatment and medication rather than prevention. However, this is slowly changing. Dr, Ryan Meili, a family physician in Saskatchewan, Canada and founder of Upstream: Institute for a Healthy Society is just one example. He states, "They (health care experts) aren't satisfied with simply pulling drowning kids out of the river; though this is obviously important, they also look upstream to ask why kids are falling in the river in the first place" (in *The Daily Courier* newspaper, March 24, 2015).

We hear in our practice all of the time patients feeling frustrated when walking down the aisles in local grocery stores trying to choose from hundreds of supplements. What is it that one really needs? We get asked that all the time. So, we have put together a list of our recommendations to cover some major deficiencies. Of course, there are going to be exceptions as everyone is unique. Another thing to consider is that you never want to treat a symptom with a supplement. You get so used to growing up with a medicine cabinet with a pill for every ailment. At the same time, you do not want to take a supplement for your headache. Rather, take a nutrient to treat a deficiency which will in turn treat the symptoms. The body will take care of itself if it has everything it needs.

Much has been written about natural versus synthetic vitamins. Do synthetic vitamins work as well as natural supplements? Does it matter what you take? It has been argued that synthetic vitamins have the same molecular structure as natural vitamins and that laboratory-created synthetic supplements have to meet rigid standards and therefore contamination is less likely. Most of the vitamins you find on the pharmacy or grocery store shelves are synthetic, chemically manufactured supplements. They are also considerably cheaper to purchase than the natural supplements and have a longer shelf life than their natural counterparts.

However, synthetic vitamins often have other additives that can adversely affect the vitamin or even be harmful to health. Synthetic vitamins, including some popular brands may be made from coal tar derivatives and may contain dyes such as Red #40, Yellow #6, Blue #6, sweeteners, or preservatives calcium disodium EDTA,BHA/BHT, chalk, sodium benzoate, dl-alpha-tocopheryl, methylcellulose, cupric sulfate, carnauba wax, silicon, titanium, petroleum derived chemical solvents such as ethyl cellulose, sugar alcohols (ethyl alcohol or erythritol), hydrogenated palm oil, hypromellose or polyvinyl and may be coated with methylene chloride, a carcinogenic material. (http://www.vitamins-nutrition.org/). Allergic reactions can include lethargy, forgetfulness sleeplessness and depression.

Natural vitamins contain multiple nutrients that synthetics do not contain. These nutrients work synergistically to enhance absorption and to enhance effectiveness.

Natural supplements are concentrated from natural sources such as plant or other natural derivatives. The manufacturing process uses no extreme heat or toxic ingredients or chemical coatings or binders or fillers that may block absorption.

It is important to choose a quality supplement from a reputable brand and to keep in mind that just because it says it's natural, does not mean it is a quality product. There are many questionable natural supplements on the market either containing ingredients not listed on the label, or not containing the ingredients in the stated amounts on the label. It is important for you to do your homework. Also, care needs to be taken when examining research related to vitamins because the research generally looks at the effectiveness of one nutrient only. The problem with this is that nutrients do not work in isolation. Rather the effectiveness depends on the interaction of the nutrient in combination of other nutrients in the body. Additionally, research studies using synthetic supplements may have totally different results from studies using natural source vitamins. Also, some studies are conducted with dosages too low to show any difference in health benefits (http://www.healthconceptsint.com). Again, we stress that it is important that you become an informed consumer and do your own research.

Whole Food MultiVitamins

Is it necessary or even safe to take a daily multivitamin such as one-a-day? When we mention whole food multivitamins, what are we talking about? What is the difference between whole food multivitamins and synthetic vitamins?

Whole food vitamin are basically just concentrated foods ground up and processed into a supplement form. Whole food based supplements have numerous enzymes and nutrients that the body uses to process and utilize the vitamins whereas synthetic multivitamins generally do not have the added enzymes and nutrients to process the vitamins it in the same way. There is some research that suggests that individuals who take a synthetic one-a-day have lower blood circulating vitamins than those who take no vitamin at all. We do not know why that is the case. They are likely to be the cheapest vitamins containing potentially harmful ingredients, and often shellac coated (http://www.naturalnews.com/036650_synthetic_vitamins_disease_side_effects.html).

The way we like to look at whole food multiple vitamins is that it is like an insurance policy. If you are eating very well, lots of raw vegetables and getting what you think you need, it is possible that there still are certain nutrients you are missing. It is a whole foods insurance policy to help prevent deficiencies. You do not have to be too concerned about overdosing from a quality whole food multiple vitamin.

Always check the labels before buying your nutritional supplements. We provide links to a number of websites at the end of the chapter where you can find whole food multivitamins as well as other natural whole food nutritional supplements.

In this next section we take a look at the four supplements that are often deficient in the average American diet.

Omega 3 Fatty Acids

Another common deficiency we have talked about previously are omega 3 fats. Americans are generally way out of the healthy ratio of omega 6 to omega 3s. Primitive culture's diets reflect 2:1. Americans are around 21:1. Too much omega 6 can create inflammation in the body and lead to increase in all diseases. Inflammation has been tied to almost every disease. It is kind of the driving force to disease. Low omega 3 levels can increase your susceptibility to inflammation and pain sensitivity. Our diets, unfortunately, are rich in omega 6s which can aggravate inflammatory pathway, while omega 3's block inflammation. The ratios are skewed, so most Americans even if they are eating a healthy diet may still be somewhat deficient in omega 3s. It is a simple thing to supplement your diet with more omega 3s, however, it is important to get a high quality omega 3 because it oxidizes very easily and some of the omega 3s on the market may be doing more harm than good. We hear people saying we don't like taking fish oils because they burp up fish and that may be because it has gone rancid.

The most important thing to look for when you are buying omega 3 is to make sure it does not smell or taste like fish. Check that it contains approximately 800 mg. EPA & 500 mg. of DHA per daily serving and that it has been tested for PCBs and mercury. Also, look for a liquid form of omega 3 in a dark glass bottle with added lemon, vitamin E or rosemary to help it from oxidizing. It is a very fragile oil sensitive to temperature. You are not going to want to leave this fish oil above the stove or in the car. It is best to store it in the fridge to keep it fresh.

Currently in the U.S. there are no laws stating you have to test for mercury or PCBs. So, if the manufacturer goes through the process of spending the money to test their product, it will be labelled on the bottle, so check for that. We both use fish oil from a company called Innate Choice (www.innatechoice.com). They get their fish oil from Norway and use a third party to test for mercury, PCB and rancidity. It is more expensive than some fish oils, but then they are spending the money to do the testing which adds to the cost. Take care when buying omega 3s from local groceries or big chain stores because it is more likely that they are going to be very poor quality fish oils and consequently they may end up doing more harm than good. So, make sure you are getting the right one. It is worth spending a few extra dollars for that.

Vitamin D3

Vitamin D deficiency is very common, more so than in the past. Vitamin D deficiency can have a multitude of symptoms such as depression, digestive issues, bone marrow health, headaches, muscle cramps, weight gain, joint and muscle pain, general weakness, restless sleep, fatigue, poor concentration, bladder problems, constipation and high blood pressure. Flu season is highest when vitamin D levels are the lowest. You will want to make sure you are getting vitamin D3 which is far superior to vitamin D2. It is of interest that a prescription for vitamin D is generally Vitamin D2 and milk is fortified with vitamin D2. It is reassuring that testing more for Vitamin D deficiency is becoming more prevalent.

Probiotics

Probiotics are health promoting live bacteria that we require for proper digestion of food and immune defense against illness promoting bacteria, viruses and fungi. It is such a strange thought that our body needs to have bacteria, but this is the bacteria that will promote natural beneficial flora in your gut to help keep pathogenic bacteria viruses out and infections at bay. If you are prone to gut issues you may have a deficiency in probiotics. The probiotics to look for need to be stabilized, from a good source and third party tested. The Innate Choice website sells a broad spectrum probiotic. It is stabilized, refrigerated and shipped in such a way that the living microorganisms will not be compromised.

It is not difficult to make your own probiotics. You can find a number of different sources by simply doing a google search. One way is to buy some Kefir starter packs and just grow your own. Kombucha is another source of probiotics and simple to make. The principal is the same as using a sourdough starter to make bread.

Magnesium

Magnesium in the body serves several important functions. Contracting and relaxing muscles, certain enzyme functions, energy production and production of protein are some of these functions. Magnesium also helps repair DNA from radiation damage and if you do not have enough magnesium, the DNA cannot be repaired. Food sources include dark green leafy vegetables, nuts, almonds, cashews, seeds. For an adult male to obtain the recommended daily requirement of 400-430 mgs. per day, he would have to eat a large quantity of leafy green vegetables to get that amount. This is not always a simple task.

As mentioned, magnesium serves an important part in muscle contraction. So, if you tend to have a lot of tight muscles, a good quality magnesium supplement may make a difference in a matter of days. We generally think of potassium when it comes to muscles, but sometimes it can be a magnesium deficiency. So, it is very important to supplement if you have some concerns about a magnesium deficiency, but a first step might be to get tested for a possible deficiency.

Prevent or Reverse Disease

When you are talking about a sufficient amount of nutrients your body needs obviously that is going to prevent disease, but at the same time we want to realize that some individuals coming into a healthy lifestyle may already have some diseases. That is a reality of life. By maintaining a healthy lifestyle - bringing your body weight down through exercise, proper nutrition and stress management you are more likely to prevent and even in some cases reverse disease. We have patients with Type 2 diabetes who have been told that they need to be on medication for their lifetime in order to manage the symptoms of the disease. Yet there are situations where individuals diagnosed with Type 2 diabetes have been able to maintain normal blood sugar levels without medication. We have personally seen someone completely insulin dependent who in the course of several months with some fairly radical lifestyle changes, more of a Paleo type of diet, lean meats, more fruits, vegetables, good healthy fats, was able to come off the insulin and eventually off the other diabetic medications. Literally lifestyle was the treatment for it. Of course, it is not going to happen overnight. The medication for diabetes is intended to just manage the disease, to manage the symptoms of the disease. These medications will manage the symptoms or the blood sugar levels, but they will not alleviate the root of the problem.

There are many chronic diseases and obviously there are multiple causes for these diseases. Many of these diseases require intensive interventions and long-term treatment plans. Some have no known cures. However, we know that deficiencies in certain nutrients can make you more prone to certain types of illnesses. For example, vitamin. D levels as they go lower increase your risk to certain types of melanoma. Other types of cancer such as colon cancer are increasing so preventing the disease again from the standpoint of a good and healthy lifestyle is obviously wise. Cancer treatments in North America are slowly changing but currently chemical therapy and radiation, the two things known to cause cancer, are the standard practice.

There are some cancer centers popping up in North America that utilize different approaches to cancer treatment. Some of these cancer centers use a combination of treatments including nutrient therapy to address cancer to try to change the physiology inside the body so that it is toxic to cancer cells. If you have cancer, we are not recommending that you do not do these types of treatments, just do some research on your own so that you are better able to make informed choices before resorting to radical treatments. If you or someone you know is undergoing chemo or radiation that seem to be the only option at this particular time, you can often include nutritional therapies along the way as well. We recommend you do your research on that.

In summary, with a healthy lifestyle – proper nutrition including beneficial fiber and whole foods, exercise, weight and stress management and quality nutritional supplements when diets are insufficient, such as fish oil, probiotics, and whole food supplements you are more likely to prevent and even reverse disease.

Thirty-Day Action Plan

Discuss with your physician about your current medical situation. How lifestyle modification may reduce your need for these medications.

We recommend you create a supplemental action plan to address any deficiencies you may have. Also, if there is some concern about disease, is there something you can do about disease reversal? Take our recommendations, download the action plan we have included and research some of the supplement companies and decide if certain vitamins, fish oils or probiotics may be beneficial for you. Download an action plan at http://thewellnesssolution.co /wp-content/uploads/2013/04/mod-5-handout.pdf.

If you buy these and put them all at the back of the drawer or cabinet behind a bunch of other stuff, you are probably not going to remember to take these. Again, keep them in a place where you are going to see them. Consistency is the key. Also, discuss with your physician about medications you are currently on and how necessary are these. If you don't have a physician who supports you in these conversations, perhaps you need to find one that does. Also, if you work with several physicians using several pharmacies, try to bring that back under your own roof again so that you don't have an overlap in medications.

Unfortunately, as we mentioned earlier, a lot of medical practitioners do not have a lot of knowledge in nutrition and supplementation so if your physician falls into that category it might be time to find someone else because nutrition can be a huge part in disease management.

Under no circumstances do we recommend that you just go cold turkey off all your medications because you are now adopting a wellness lifestyle. This is something you are going to want to speak to your physician about and talk about reducing or taking yourself off the medications. Often just a simple lifestyle modification can change things quickly. You have to realize that getting off some of these medications can create some withdrawal effects so it is very important to work with someone who is qualified to help through the transition. You never just want to go cold turkey off medications such as anti-depressants. You want to reduce it over time with medical supervision. A good physician will work with you in those areas. If you need to shop around a bit, we recommend you do that.

Chapter 6

The Hidden Truth about Diet and Nutrition

In the first part of this chapter we will discuss concerns related to the current state of health in the United States and the second part makes recommendations as to foods you should be eating or eliminating to help you to become healthier.

"Let food be your medicine and medicine be your food." Hippocrates

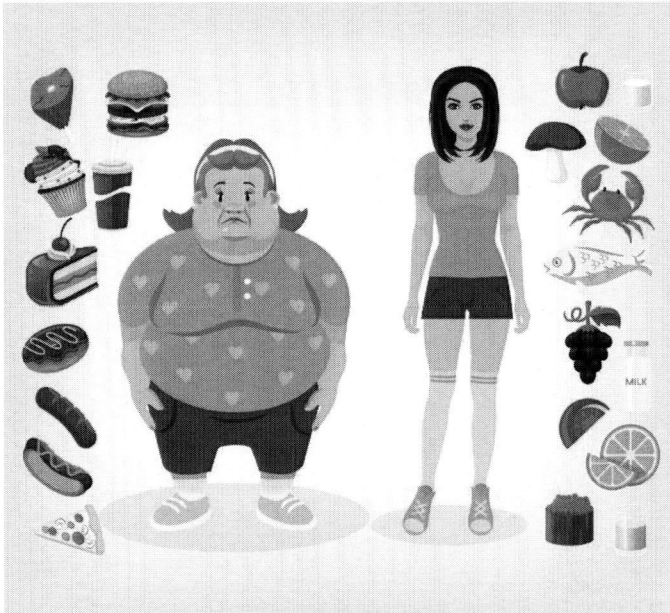

In this chapter, we look at what is meant by a good diet and some of the conflicting information surrounding diets. We will examine what we should be eating and not eating and the research behind our recommendations. After reading this chapter you will better understand why Hippocrates said, "Let food be your medicine and medicine be your food."

In the United States, the rates of obesity and diseases such as Type 2 diabetes, heart disease and cancer are on the rise. These diseases are partly based in lifestyle choices, specifically in diet and consequently may be preventable. The two diseases particularly on the rise are Type 2 diabetes and obesity. Before we address these topics in more depth, we will briefly recap the last five chapters. We have covered a lot of material in the previous chapters so it is helpful to highlight some of the key points before proceeding. It is also beneficial to go back and review the material with a fresh set of eyes. When you take on new information often things you have read in the past can take on a new perspective as well.

Obesity Epidemic

More than one-third of American adults are obese.

http://www.cdc.gov/obesity/data/adult.html

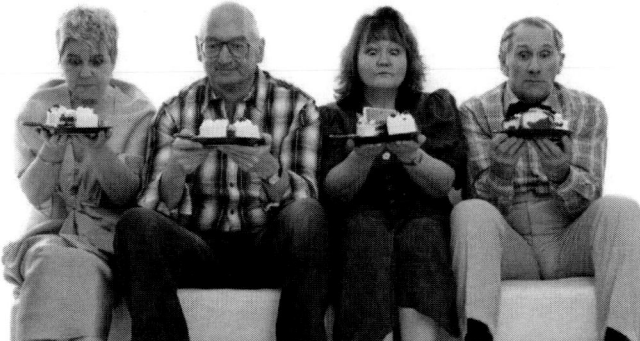

Obesity is a disease that can lead to chronic conditions such as Type 2 diabetes, heart disease, high blood pressure, gall bladder disease, sleep apnea, mobility issues and even some forms of cancer. Various criteria have been used over the years to define obesity in the United States. In general terms, obesity can be described as an excessive accumulation of body fat to the extent where the person's health may be adversely impacted. Particularly concerning is abdominal fat which has been linked to greater mortality than body fat elsewhere. Body mass index (BMI) and waist circumference have often been used as a simple index to categorize overweight or obesity adults. To determine BMI, a person's weight is divided by the square of the person's height (http://www.who.int/mediacentre/factsheets/fs311/en/).

Of Americans, as a whole, just 35 percent are considered to be of normal weight. The Food Research and Action Center (FRAC) notes that obesity rates in the United States have doubled between the 1970s and 2009 with 68.5% of adults, 31.8% of children and adolescents considered overweight (http://frac.org/initiatives/hunger-and-obesity/obesity-in-the-us/). Focusing specifically on obesity, a 2013 Gallup poll cites obesity rates at 27.1 percent, the highest measured by Gallop since 2008 when it first started tracking obesity rates in the United States (http://www.foxnews.com/health/2014/05/22/us-obesity-rate-reaches-new-high/)

It is of interest that Colorado with 21.3% has the lowest number of obese people in the United States with the fittest in all of North America being in Boulder where a mere 12.4% were classified as obese. Boulder even beat the fittest Canadian city where the overall obesity rate is 17%.

On the other end of the obesity spectrum is West Virginia with a rate of 35.1%, with Huntington ranking the highest in the country with almost 40% of its population considered obese (http://stateofobesity.org/states/wv/; http://www.telegraph.co.uk/news/worldnews/northamerica/usa/10751039/Huntington-West-Virginia-named-fattest-US-town-as-obesity-rate-rises.html).

Looking specifically at children, a comparative study by the U.S. Centers for Disease Control and Prevention notes that approximately 17.5% of American children between the ages of 3 to 19 are obese, compared to 13% of Canadian children the same age (in http://health.usnews.com/healthnews/articles/2015/08/25/american-kids-growing-fatter-than-their-canadian-cousins).

Although the overall number of obese people in Canada is less than the United States, obesity rates in Canada have also increased with a current obesity rate of approximately 18.3% (http://globalnews.ca/news/1186942/nova-scotians-among-the-most-overweight-obese-in-canada-cmaj/; http://www.vancouver sun.com/health/Obesity+rates+higher+than+previous+report+still+lowest+Canada+StatsCan/9888839/story.html).

British Columbia has the lowest rate of obesity in Canada with 19%, while the city of Kelowna in BC is the fittest with 17% obesity. At the other end of the spectrum, the province of Nova Scotia at 37.5 per cent is the least fit with the city of Saint John, New Brunswick having the dubious honor of being the highest in the nation with 38.1% obesity. (http://www.foxnews.com/health/2014/05/22/us-obesity-rate-reaches-new-high/).

Healthy lifestyle choices are the key to preventing and reversing obesity. It is of concern that the most obese places in the United States are primarily lower-income, blue-collar areas where lifestyle habits are less healthy than in the northern and western states (http://www.cdc.gov/obesity/data/adult.html).

Changing poor, entrenched lifestyle habits can be difficult, but it is possible with increased awareness of what constitutes healthy lifestyle choices, it is possible for every American to improve their overall health and longevity. Our aim by writing this chapter is to contribute towards that objective.

Below are some sites for further research on this topic:

- Centers for Disease Control and Prevention (CDC): http://www.cdc.gov/

- Canadian Community Health Survey (CCHS): http://www23.statcan.gc.ca/imdb/p2SV.pl?Function=getSurvey&SDDS=3226
- Endocrine Society (ISC): http://obesityinamerica.org/statistics/
- International Association for the Study of Obesity (IASO): www.healthinfonet.ecu.edu.au/key-resources/organisations?oid=645
- National Institute of Diabetes and Digestive and Kidney Disease (NIDDK): http://www.niddk.nih.gov/health-information/health-communication-programs/win/Pages/default.aspx
- The American Obesity Association (AOA): http://obesity.procon.org
- The World Health Organization (WHO): http://www.who.int/gho/publications/world_health_statistics/en/

Diabetes Epidemic

29 million people in the United States (9.3%) have diabetes.

(http://www.cdc.gov/Features/DiabetesFactSheet/)

At the outset, it is important to distinguish between Type 1 and Type 2 diabetes. There is no known way to prevent Type 1 diabetes, while most cases of Type 2 diabetes can be prevented by appropriate lifestyle choices. Both forms of diabetes can develop at any age. At present one out of three Americans will develop Type 2 diabetes. The statistics are similar in Canada with approximately one in three people affected by 2020.

Type 2 diabetes, which is often connected to being inactive and overweight, can be prevented and generally reversed with healthy lifestyle changes. On the other hand, there is no known cure for Type 1 diabetes, however Type 1 diabetics are often fit and health conscious because the diabetes has not been brought on by poor lifestyle choices and they are aware of the necessity to maintain a healthy diet and regular exercise schedule. Currently, promising clinical trials for reversing Type 1 diabetes are being conducted. Of the 29 million people in the United States with diabetes, only 5% are Type 1.

Controlling blood sugar levels is crucial for all diabetics. This can be addressed with a healthy lifestyle, specifically by a healthy diet and regular exercise schedule. There might be some genetic predisposition, particularly with Type 1 diabetes. However, if you have a healthy lifestyle it doesn't mean you are going to get the disease just because someone in your family had it. Type 2 diabetes is definitely preventable and reversible. There is a misconception that if grandma or grandpa had diabetes or if it's in your family, you are going to get it. It can be a predisposition but if you eat a good healthy diet you will be less likely to have to deal with Type 2 diabetes.

In August 2005 Franz Scholz, et al. published an article in *Nature* suggesting a connection between alcohol tolerance and hangovers. (http://www.nature.com/nature/journal/v436/n7052/abs/nature03864.html)

The researchers used fruit flies as their subjects and they did not conclude that humans had a hangover gene. It was the popular press who publicized the catchy title and suggested a link. However, for the purposes of stressing our point, let us assume that you had a hangover gene and therefore you had increased susceptibility to hangovers. However, if you do not drink alcohol, you are not going to get a hangover. So, it does not matter if you have the gene or not.

Often, when we look at genetics it can steal a lot of our power if we allow it to. "Oh, I have this gene so I am destined for this." Thus, it takes away our personal power and then we are just at the mercy of our genetics. "I will throw in my hat and will just live my life because there is not much I can do". This could not be further from the truth. Knowing that we have a genetic predisposition to a disease should encourage us more to health and wellness because our genetics have not changed in thousands of years, but our lifestyles and diets certainly have and that is where we are starting to see these diseases come out. So, if we could go back to a better type of lifestyle like we had thousands of years ago, we might see many of these diseases go away again.

What Should We Be Eating

It is possible to reverse many lifestyle diseases.

126

When we talk about diet and nutrition, a common question is what is it that we should be eating? There is a lot of controversy regarding this topic and we will address this further in the following chapters. One of our main goal with the wellness solution is to try to dispel a lot of the myths, a lot of the controversies and just to get down to the nuts and bolts as to what is true health and wellness. Our current disease state has a lot to do with our lifestyle, so if we look at a healthier lifestyle and try to emulate what that is then that should get us closer to what we should be eating.

Cultures several thousand years ago ate primarily meats, fruits and vegetables - unprocessed whole foods. These foods were obviously not something with a food label or in a box, often with numerous additives and chemicals. So, if we could just clean up our diet and get back to basic whole foods that people were eating in the past compared to what people are eating now it would go a long way to staying healthy. Of course, with the marvel of modern medicine we are now living longer than ever before even with all the processed foods, but the quality of life is not necessarily there.

There are a number of more recent books, such as Dan Buettner's *Blue Zone* (2015) and Eric Plasker's *The Hundred Year Lifestyle* (2007) that examine the relationship between healthy longevity and lifestyle. There is general agreement that there is a correlation between healthy longevity regular exercise, an encouraging social network, ability to manage stress effectively, and a primarily whole food diet.

We are definitely living longer, but the quality of life is atrocious. If the last 20-30 years is to be lived with Type 2 diabetes, obesity, osteoarthritis, sleep apnea or cancer treatments, then the last years of your life may not be well lived. You may have longevity because modern medicine can keep you alive, but you will not have the quality to enjoy your life to the fullest. Vaccines, antibiotics and other advances in medicine have significantly reduced mortality rates and increased longevity, but what is reducing our quality of life or killing us is primarily how we live.

Our genetic code has not changed all that much in 10,000 years, but there are drastic lifestyle changes and there is no way for genetics to catch up to that. Our genes and our bodies right now, for example, have no concept of what to do with high fructose corn syrup which is wreaking havoc in our bodies. So, the conversation should not be so much on living longer, but rather on living a long, healthy and purposeful life. If you knew you were going to live to be a 100 years old or beyond, what changes would you make to your lifestyle now to ensure a healthier life? Make the decision now.

It is possible to reverse many lifestyle diseases. The body is designed for that. It has most of what it needs to get there - it just needs the right equation to get there. Manage your stress, cultivate and maintain positive friendships and social networks, eat a healthy primarily whole food diet, get sufficient sleep and drink enough water. Much of this is just basic stuff we already know, but you have to do it consistently. So, if you live to be a 100 or beyond, you will want to be active doing the things you want to do which is very possible.

We hear every day in our practice older patients coming up with different complaints, with different ailments that they just chalk up to old age. This attitude is just throwing in the hat and not taking responsibility for improving their own health. They just assume that their sleep apnea, brittle bones or arthritis are an inevitable consequence of old age. That is not necessarily the case. Arthritis is driven by inflammation which in turn is driven by stress and diet which happens over the course of decades.

So, make the decision now to improve your lifestyle bit by bit every day. Be determined to be the best you can be today and every day. If you just try to do a little bit better each day, there may be a couple of vices you may want to hold on to for a couple of months, but as long as you start adding good things, bad things will slowly fade away.

Problem with the Food Pyramid

We have given the food pyramid a bad rap in the past and we are going to do the same now. It has gone through a lot of change over the years. Following its creation in 1992, the food pyramid ended up being stagnant and not well used for a number of years. It had grown dated, somewhat confusing and cumbersome to use. So, in 2005 the federal government released an updated version titled My Pyramid, which unfortunately many considered equally confusing.

Then in June 2011, My Plate replaced My Pyramid. The change was spearheaded by First Lady Michelle Obama to help combat obesity by encouraging parents to help their children make healthier dietary choices (www.cnpp.usda.gov/sites/default/files/myplate_miplato/PressRelease.pdf). Our original concern with the food pyramid was that much of the data was based on old research. Some of these studies came out decades ago.

As an example, they had compared wheat flour to white flour and they found that the white flour produced more disease than the wheat flour. Rather than saying the wheat flour also produced diseases they said let us promote that as a healthier food. In fact, both of them were bad. White flour was just worse.

In 1928, the Republican Party promised a chicken in every pot if Herbert Hoover won the election. The guarantee of cheaper food for every Americans was, of course, as appealing then as it is now. So, how do you get cheaper food for everyone? Accordingly, what came about was that they eventually subsidized crops such as soybeans, corn, and wheat (http://www.downsizinggovernment. org/agriculture/subsidies).

The problem is that these foods are all carbohydrate rich foods and not necessarily rich in nutrition. The Physicians Committee for Responsible Medicine states "the U.S. Department of Agriculture (USDA) supports agricultural producers through a variety of programs that tend to favor, either directly or indirectly, the production of unhealthy foods that are implicated in the diseases that have steadily increased over the decades and now impose a significant burden on Americans" (http://www.pcrm.org/ health/reports/agriculture-and-health-policies-unhealthful-foods). It follows that since these foods are being subsidized, a good way to promote and encourage their consumption is to include them in the food pyramid.

Also, other factors to consider are influential heavily lobbied industries, such as dairy. The dairy industry has contributed millions of dollars over the years to supportive political candidates (http://www.opensecrets.org/industries/indus.php?ind=A04++). Anytime that happens, things end up not necessarily being in the best interest for the consumer. An increasing number of health professionals and health organizations are asking whether dairy in every meal is necessary or even recommended.

The Harvard School of Public Health Nutrition Source in a recent article questions whether "dairy products are the best source of calcium for most people" (http://www.hsph.harvard.edu/nutritionsource/what-should-you-eat/calcium-and-milk/). There are numerous calcium rich foods such as salmon, sardines, bok choy, almonds, figs, leafy vegetables such as kale, spinach and collard greens. However, moderate consumptions of fermented dairy products, such as live-culture, unsweetened yogurt and Kiefer and easy to digest cheese products such gut-friendly Quark, whey cheese and curd cheese from free-range, grass-fed cows and goats are options as they are rich in gut-friendly bacteria.

The revised 2005 food pyramid has received a cross section of criticism from various health professionals and organizations over the years. In addition to the concerns related to the over-emphasis on dairy products, Harvard Nutrition Source noted that the food pyramid placed equal importance on unhealthy proteins such as processed meats as it did on healthy proteins, such as nuts, fish, poultry, and beans (http://www.hsph.harvard.edu/nutrition source/mypyramid-problems/).

The food plate icon introduced in 2011 provided a bit more clarity, however, there continues to be concerns. Dr. Mercola notes that healthy fats such as animal-based omega 3s are not mentioned. The health benefits of full fat raw dairy is totally ignored as is the mention of the dangers of trans fats which are widely consumed in America. Dr. Mercola also cautions that half of the plate consists of fruits and vegetables which is concerning since fruits are high in fructose. Also, there should be some mention of the importance of eating organic when possible because many fruits, vegetables, beans, and grains may contain dangerous pesticides.   (http://articles.mercola.com/sites/articles/archive/2011/06/23/new-food-pyramid-changes-to-less-grains-more-veggies.aspx).

The average American consumes approximately 165 pounds of sugar annually.

(http://www.webmd.com/diet/the-hidden-ingredient-that-can-sabotage-your-diet).

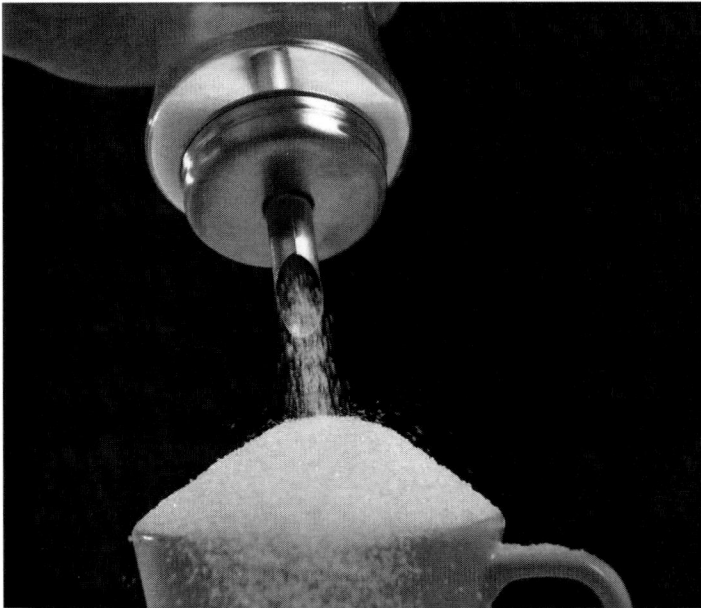

There are significant concerns related to the increasing excessive consumption of sugar. John Casey in an article on WebMD notes that the average American consumes approximately 165 pounds of sugar annually (http://www.webmd.com/diet/the-hidden-ingredient-that-can-sabotage-your-diet). Bray, et al (2004) in the American Journal of Clinical Nutrition reported that "the consumption of HFCS increased by 1000% between 1970 and 1990, far exceeding the changes in intake of any other food or food group" (http://ajcn.nutrition.org/content/79/4/537.full). It is no wonder obesity in America has reached endemic proportions.

Processed foods are loaded with added sugar, mainly high fructose corn syrup which is approximately 20% sweeter than cane sugar. Most soft drinks, juices, packaged cereals, crackers, ice cream, pastries, baked goods, jams, canned and dried fruit, condiments, processed meats, sauces, salad dressings and snack foods such as pretzels, potato chips contain large amounts high fructose corn syrup, as well as artificial flavors. Even foods touted as healthy and natural such as flavored yogurts, energy drinks, and peanut butter are often loaded with sugar. Also, be wary of low-fat foods which are often full of sugar.

We should be concerned. Not only does increased consumption of sugar lead to obesity, it can trigger health issues such as increased blood pressure and cholesterol, insulin resistance, mineral deletion, arthritis and liver disease. Dr. Mercola notes that even infant formula can contain as much sugar as one can of pop (http://www.mercola.com/infographics/fructose-overload.htm).

Whenever possible look for food options containing less sugar. There are healthier options for an increasing number of food products. Read the labels, purchase fresh produce, meats and fish, preferably organic. When that's not an option, buy frozen or water-packed canned foods in glass containers. Buy grass-fed rather than grain-fed. If you want to fatten up a cow, you feed them grains. So, at the end of the day, grains are carbohydrates which basically is sugar.

The body turns carbohydrates into sugar. A single slice of bread made from 100% whole wheat grains has a higher glycemic index than 1 tsp of table sugar, so basically you are just eating sugar. There are also healthier choices for condiments such as ketchup that aren't loaded with high fructose corn syrup. Of course, you may need to look a bit harder to find them.

When you read the labels, look at the list of additives. There are a number of fruits and vegetables you should buy organic because of the pesticides. There are a number of lists on various sites provided by organizations such as the Environmental Working Group (http://www.ewg.org/foodnews/summary.php) and the David Suzuki Foundation (http://www.davidsuzuki.org/what-you-can-do/queen-of-green/faqs/food/what-are-the-dirty-dozen-and-the-clean-fifteen/).

The Perfect Human Diet

Is there such a thing as a perfect human diet suitable for everyone?

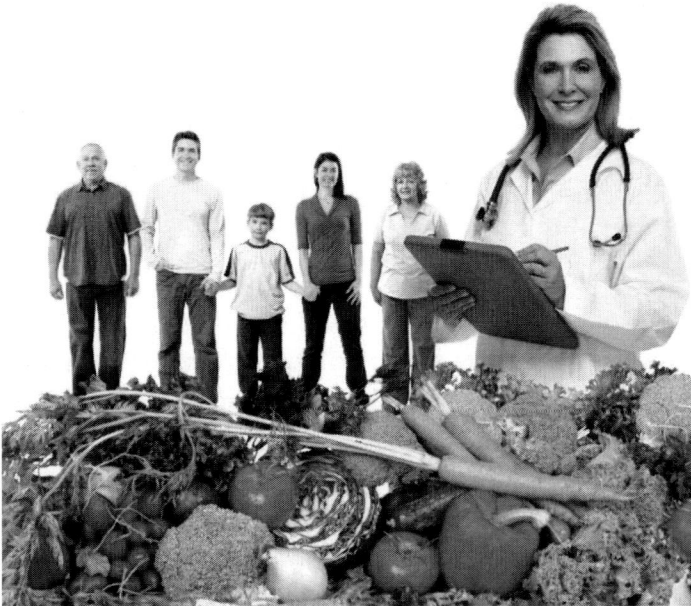

Is there such a thing as a perfect human diet suitable for everyone? Are we not all different? There is so much contradictory advice it is hard to know what to believe. Recommendations as to what to eat and not to eat seem to be continually changing. Yesterday, butter, chocolate, coffee and red wine were *bad* and today they are *good*. Is it any wonder that people are becoming increasingly skeptical? Best-selling books such as *The Hundred Year Lifestyle* (Eric Plasker, 2007), *The Paleo Diet* (Loren Cordain, 2010), *Wheat Belly* (William Davis, 2012), *Perfect Health Diet: Regain Health and Lose Weight by Eating the Way You Were Meant to Eat* (Paul Jaminet ,2013); *Brain Maker* (David Perlmutter, 2015) and *Blue Zones* (Dan Buettner, 2015) seem to be advocating different advice as to what to eat and not to eat in order to maintain or achieve health and longevity.

Cordain, in his *Paleo Diet*, recommends avoiding all dairy, grains, gluten, legumes and processed foods. Jaminet's *Perfect Health Diet* is similar to the *Paleo Diet*, but permits rice, potatoes and full-fat dairy, but not non-fat or low-fat. Cordain and Jaminet say not to eat legumes, wheat or dairy, but the other authors give approval to legumes and dairy with some restrictions. Davis similarly advocates no wheat products, but permits legumes and non-gluten grains. Cordain, Jaminet, Pearlmutter, Davis, all give a thumbs up to full-fat foods, while Plasker and Buettner recommend low-fat as the best option.

On the surface the recommendations appear contradictory. However, if we delve a bit deeper as to what they have to say, there are commonalities with the bulk of their recommendations. Let's look briefly at the commonalities we can all agree on as to what we should eat or not eat in order to gain and maintain healthy lifestyles and longevity.

A number of supporters of *The Paleo Diet,* such as Paul Jaminet and Chris Kresser, author of *Are Legumes "Paleo"? And Does It Really Matter?* (2014, in http://chriskresser.com/are-legumes-paleo) appear to view the Paleo diet as more of a broad template, rather than as a prescriptive diet. For example, when it comes to beans they appear to support the thinking of high profile media personalities such as Drs. Oz and Rozen, who recommend beans such as lentils, garbanzo and pinto to lower blood sugar levels and blood pressure levels, and the risk of heart disease. They further state that beans will help reduce belly fat and to protect the cells from oxidation damage. (Beans are brilliant for blood, heart and belly, B4, *The Province*, Dec. 30, 2012; *RealAge.com*; twitter.com/YoungDrMike). Of course, beans do not factor into a purist interpretation of Cordain's *Paleo Diet*.

There are also commonalities as to what not to eat: packaged cereals, refined sugar and high fructose corn syrup, processed foods, refined vegetable oils, candy and salty or sugary snack foods, grain-fed, hormone and antibiotic injected meat and poultry, farmed fish are some of these.

Common healthy foods include grass-fed, hormone and antibiotic free meats, non-farmed, mid-size fish, fresh organic fruits and vegetables, berries, free-range organic eggs, nuts and seeds, again, preferably organic, healthy oils, such as olive, coconut and flax and fermented foods. Also, most of these authors consider a limited consumption of dark chocolate, red wine, sweet potatoes, rice, some legumes, and coffee and tea, including fermented kombucha tea, as healthy. However, care needs to be exercised when consuming legumes because a large per cent are genetically modified and they can be toxic in their raw state. Limited consumption of full-fat, non-homogenized, grass-fed dairy, particularly Kieffer and yogurt and cheeses such as Kurd and whey cheese, dairy alternatives such as coconut and almond milk and fermented vegetables and eggs are considered healthy.

The Perfect Human Diet: Our Recommendations

"The routine use of antibiotics in farming is contributing to the rise of antibiotic resistant bacteria, so once easy to treat infections are becoming more serious even deadly". Consumer Report, Oct. 2015

New discoveries and new research findings related to health, nutrition and the foods that we eat are being made on an on-going basis. Based on the information we have at present, we do have recommendations as to what constitutes an ideal diet.

We support the Paleo diet in principal as a basic starting point or template. Eating organic, unprocessed, non-GMO whole foods, free-range, grass-fed meat, wild-caught fish or shellfish, free-range eggs and poultry, nuts and seeds, leafy green vegetables, berries and fruit, fermented foods such as fermented vegetables and fermented dairy such as Kieffer and yogurt.

Dairy should be organic, full-fat, non-homogenized from free-range, grass-fed, antibiotic, hormone free cows or goats. Similarly, meats should be free range, grass fed, hormone and antibiotic free. Venison, such as elk or deer would be a good option. They are not eating corn or soy, nor have they been fed by-products of other animals, or been injected with antibiotics and growth hormones. They have lived relatively happy lives grazing freely. So, these types of meats are going to be your best and ultimately that is what nature intended. It is alarming to learn that conventional beef in feed lots may be fed chicken coop waste, remains of pigs and chicken and even plastic pellets and candy.

Also concerning are the hormones and antibiotics and other drugs given to conventional cows. In the October 2015 issue,

Consumer Report warns that "the routine use of antibiotics in farming is contributing to the rise of antibiotic resistant bacteria, so once easy to treat infections are becoming more serious even deadly". The Report also highlights the concern that the American beef industry is controlled by five powerful beef lobbies who are resistant to changing their precarious practices (http://www. consumerreports.org/cro/magazine/2015/10/index.htm).

Stay clear of farmed fish which can contain high concentrations of antibiotics, pesticides and even color (http:// articles.mercola.com/sites/articles/archive/2013/07/09/farmed-salmon-dangers.aspx). As for shellfish, it is unfortunate we are starting to see more and more contaminates with toxic oceans. It is worrisome that with the scramble for ever-increasing profits, the use of antibiotics in aquaculture and farming is increasing. You will pay more for wild salmon, free-range beef and chicken not fed hormones or antibiotics, but in terms of your overall health, it is worth the extra costs.

Chicken and free range organic eggs produced by chickens able to run around and not cooped up in tiny pens are going to be healthier. Anytime you take any species of animals and put them in a small area, you are going to create stress and unhealthier animals. You will pay more for chicken that has been raised in more space to run around, but that chicken is going to be a lot healthier and the meat is going to taste so much superior.

Then again, this is going to be a superior diet. For those people who have philosophical reasons not to eat meat, we respect that. And we appreciate that there are ways to eat healthy without eating meat. Many people assume meats are unhealthy, but it's more about the way the animal is raised and fed and how the meat is processed, than the meat itself. The adage you are what you eat, is the animal. If the animal is not eating properly if they are living a stressful life, if they are fed hormones, antibiotics, by-products from other animals, plastic pellets, candy, soy and grains, the tissue and fat is going to be different.

You can have an organic egg but if it says grain fed on the cover it is going to be lacking healthy omega 3s and things like that. And if it says omega 3, they may be adding inferior omega 3. So, free range is going to be eating what the chickens were designed to eat and in general it is going to be much healthier.

As for fruits and vegetables, the best scenario would be to eat organic, but again if that is cost prohibitive or if you are just starting out, use our list of recommendations from the EWG site (http://www.ewg.org/ foodnews/dirty_dozen_list.php). The site lists the top dozen worst pesticide laden vegetables and fruit and the cleanest fifteen (http://www.ewg.org/foodnews/clean_fifteen _list.php). Celery, apples, strawberries are among the worst. These are the places to start and the thicker-skinned things that can be peeled are not quite as bad.

With nuts and seeds you want to make sure they are organic and not processed. We do not recommend peanuts, which are a legume, because peanuts have a high susceptibility to contaminants such as Aflatoxin which has been associated liver disease. Some people also have serious allergies to peanuts. Of course, in countries in Africa, peanuts are a staple. It is worth mention that aflatoxins, but to a much less extent, have also been found in nuts such as walnuts and pecans, as well as in soybeans, grains, spices and dairy. When nuts are processed, you are going to add a lot of oils and salt which are not the best for you. Unprocessed nuts are going to be far superior to an oiled salted roasted one. You can find them in a refrigerated section of a store. As well, they are going to be healthier, so if a nut or seed has been sitting on the shelf for a long time the oils in it are going to be oxidized and perhaps rancid as well. Limit your consumption of nuts because the nuts are a concentrated source of calories.

Also, limit your consumption of dairy. Contrary to previous beliefs, fat can be healthy. We need fat but it must be the healthy non-processed types.

Recently HHS and USDA updated their recommendations on fat consumption removing a restriction on healthy unsaturated fats. These will be released later in 2015 (http://health.gov /dietaryguidelines/2015/). Restrict grains to primarily gluten-free, non-GMO modified. Similarly restrict legumes and soy to non-GMO. Consider making your own sour dough bread if you crave breads. Restrict or eliminate wherever possible, the condiments, the refined foods, the sodas, fruit juices, packaged cereals and products sweetened with high fructose corn syrup. Most vegetables you can eat in unlimited quantities.

So, to recap our list of foods to avoid, obviously your junk food, packaged, processed foods, things designed to sit on the shelf for 3 to 6 months or even longer, your Twinkies, the candy bars, few exceptions like your super dark chocolate 70% or higher would be a good option for something to eat in moderation. Chocolate is good for you because it has a lot of antioxidants, but your sugar filled milk chocolate is something to avoid. Of course, you have to realize 70% chocolate is still 30% sugar.

For myself, I found that the benefit of the dark chocolate is that it is difficult to eat large quantities because it is so rich. So, for me, one little snap of the end satisfies my chocolate craving without eating the whole bar. Your condiments, such as ketchup, in moderation, is not going to be a big deal if it is only an occasional, minor part of your diet. Potato chips, things that are heavily oiled and salted especially the trans fats, artificially hydrogenated oils that have a long shelf life, all those you will want to avoid.

Also, dairy in moderation is not a big deal but in excess it can be a problem. Wheat can be problematic. According to Davis in *Wheat Belly*, the wheat we have now is nothing like the wheat we had 100-200 years ago. It is hybridized to such a point the gluten particles are becoming an issue. Your grains and corn are often genetically modified, however non-GMO corn and grains are becoming more readily available with increased consumer demand.

Action Plan

For an action plan, we ask you to identify several areas you would like to change or clean up. What are the first steps you would like to take? Whether it is reducing your wheat intake or sugar-laden packaged cereals or researching where you can purchase hormone and antibiotic-free organic grass-fed beef. Perhaps you can locate freezer packs of free range, grass-fed beef directly from a ranch for a reasonable price. Grass-fed antibiotic-free beef in the stores can be pricy.

So, decide what your priorities will be. Decide that maybe this month you will give up diet soda as your first big change. It does not have to be revolutionary to your health. So, use that worksheet. Think what those things are going to be. Do not feel you have to make these changes overnight. Just proceed a step at a time. With this action plan start making these changes. Simply focus on how to move in a positive direction towards increased health and wellness rather than staying stagnant or going the other way.

Again, we do recommend you continue to review the previous chapters. Go through some previous worksheets. If you fall off the wagon and you are not doing some of those things do not make judgement over that, just go back and start implementing those things again. Wellness never truly arrives - it is always a process of growing and changing and adapting what you do.

Chapter 7

Detoxifying Your Body

Detoxification is a simple way to get rid of the sledge in your body.

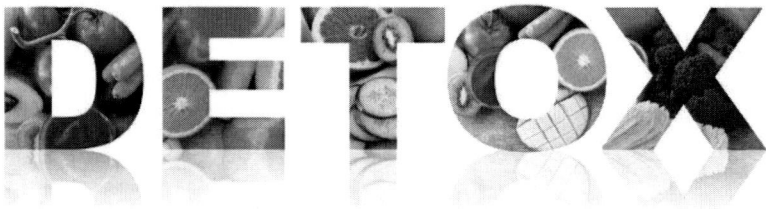

In this seventh chapter, we look at why it is important to periodically cleanse your body of toxins. We discuss how the body can become toxic and why a proper body cleanse can jumpstart your health and wellness. We will give you the most up-to-date scientific approach to the body cleanse with instructions on how to go about it and how often. We will examine why many nutritional deficiencies can start due to a slow and sluggish liver, kidney and intestinal system, why acid-alkaline balance is important in health and why it is hard for some to lose weight, while others can do it in their sleep.

We present a simple to follow purification program to assist you to cleanse your body of toxins. You develop a lot of sludge in your body that you want to get rid of. It is a lot like changing the oil in your car. So, this is a great way to do that. This program, although simple to follow, does require you to change your diet fairly radically for twenty-one days in order to detoxify your body, to reset your PH and to change your biochemistry.

There are a number of ways you can detoxify your body. We have looked at some different programs. The program we present is something you can do at home without the necessity of incurring any additional expense. Although it is not necessary to buy any special products, there are high quality pre-packaged purification kits that can be purchased from reputable companies, such as Standard Process (http://www.standardprocess.com/Standard-Process/Purification-Program#.VjFX2fmrTIU). However, they only sell to qualified health care professionals, so you will need to contact your health care provider if you wish to purchase a kit.

If you have never done a cleanse before, it is never too late to start. It can be a big change if this is your first cleanse. As far as frequency goes, we would recommend doing a cleanse at least once a year. We typically do one twice each year. Your level of toxicity can vary from location to location. If you are living in a very urban area, you may be exposed to a lot more pollution than a rural environment.

Patient Testimonials

"Two roads diverged in a wood and I took the one less travelled by and that has made all the difference"
Robert Frost, *The Road Not Taken*

Before we delve into the nitty gritty, we would like to share several testimonials of patients who have completed the twenty-one day cleanse. There were some remarkable results. We will look at some of the lab work that was done, some of the cholesterol scores and some of the dramatic changes in triglyceride levels. Some of the changes were quite astonishing.

Patient DW: *My wife and I finished our detox last Monday and have not felt this good in twenty years. We have more energy during the day and I finally get that restful sleep at night. Rarely do I wake up at 2:00 am and not get back to sleep until about 4:00 am. We have been telling all of our friends and family about this program and many of them have noticed the change in our weight and energy levels and ask how we did it. I lost about fifteen pounds and my wife lost ten pounds. We have also made changes to our regular diets. We don't remember vegetables ever tasting so good. One thing though, we miss our shakes. Thanks for your program.*

Patient SW: *I just got the results back from my physical that I took at the end of my twenty-one day detoxification program. Not only is my blood pressure back down where it needs to be, my cholesterol to the point that my doctor has taken me off both medications. I have been on blood pressure pills for five years. I didn't think it was possible to get off medication at this point. The doctor told me that whatever I am doing to keep it up.*

Today is September 13th, 2006. I started the cleanse on July 24, 2006. You told me it would change my life and you were right and I know this is just the beginning to enjoying optimum health. The changes I have already experienced are: clearer thinking (I was always in a state of overwhelm and felt like I was in a fog.); greater energy levels (Before the detox, I didn't have much energy after about 2 pm and I needed a nap every afternoon.); mental and emotional sense of well-being. I actually get excited about life. I can play with my granddaughter and actually do other things at the same time. It is unbelievable.); physical improvements (Before detoxification, I always experienced swelling in my feet, ankles and hands. After detox I have had little or no swelling at the end of the day. I have also been able to get off three prescription pills. I no longer need Nexium. Before detox if I missed Nexium after about three days my acid reflux would be bad. I thought I was having a heart attack. I rarely experience any indigestion now. But the few times I have, I have taken Zypan and in a few minutes I am fine. I have also been able to get off Ativan for anxiety and

Premarin for HRT and replace that with a woman's multi-supplement. So far everything feels great.

I have not been in a fast food restaurant for eight weeks. I have only eaten out three times since I started the program. Before the detox I ate out five to seven times each week. If you told me this would happen I would never have believed it. The best thing about this is that I haven't wanted to. My cravings are down by approximately 95 per cent. It is unbelievable. I know there are lots of things I have forgotten to mention, like no more constipation. My bowels move nearly every time I eat. I have also lost fourteen pounds, most of which was body fat. I haven't lost any lean muscle. I know I have a long way to go but I am very thankful to you that you showed me the road less travelled and with your support I will be able to continue on this road toward maximum health and fitness. All my thanks.

Patient CM: *I wanted to inform you about how my life has changed since my detoxification. You told me it would but I was skeptical at best. I was at a point where I felt I had no life. I was exhausted, constantly in pain, depressed because I couldn't lose weight. I was taking approximately 50 to 70 extra strength Tylenol and 40 to 50 Excedrin every other week because my joints hurt so badly. I would literally come home from work every day, sit in my chair and fall asleep there, sometimes not getting up until the next day. All that changed the first week I was on the detox. For the first time in years I slept soundly throughout the night. Not that fretful, restless sleep, but deep, solid sleep all night long. My ankles and hands stopped swelling, my headaches went away and I had unbelievable energy. I felt like the fog in my head had lifted and I could think more clearly. I now come home from work, cook a heathy dinner, spend quality time with my teenage daughter. I am now actively involved with extra-curricular activities and even have the energy to exercise. I no longer take any pain medication. I mean nothing. I do not need my prescription diuretics and I lost*

25 pounds in three weeks. I have continued to maintain this healthy lifestyle since the purification and I feel better than I have in the last ten years. Thank you for the opportunity to feel great and to live my life again.

Patient MC:
Test Results before Detoxification and 29 Days After
Before: Cholesterol 344   After: 162
Before: triglycerides: 787   After: 108
Before: Heart Risk: 5.5   After: 5.0

Patient JH:
Test Results before Detoxification and 22 Days After
Before: Cholesterol 230   After: 176
Before: triglycerides: 128   After: 87
Before: Heart Risk: 4.2   After: 3.8

Patient X:
Test Results before Detoxification and 27 Days After
Before: Cholesterol 231   After: 185
Before: triglycerides: 145   After: 85
Before: Heart Risk: 7.2   After: 3.7

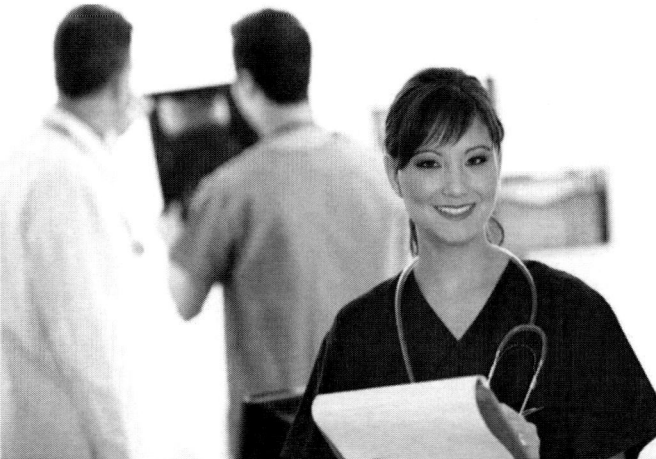

Why Are We so Toxic?

"Our children enter the world with more than 200 chemicals in their body."

CNN Series, Toxic America, 2010

Why are we so toxic? Our environment, our diet, and our medications all contribute to our toxicity. As we mentioned earlier, the levels of toxicity can vary from area to area. Individuals raised in urban environments generally have a much higher risk for developing asthma than people living in urban environments. However, regardless of our environment, we cannot get away from toxicity anymore. Therefore, it is very important to do a periodic purification.

A 100-gram portion of sugar can significantly reduce the capacity of white blood cells to engulf bacteria or cancer cells. (http://ajcn.nutrition.org/content/26/11/1180.abstract)

The CNN video series, *Toxic America* raises alarms about the staggering amount of chemical additives in our foods. The series notes, "Our children enter the world with more than 200 chemicals in their body" and that the average person in the United States consumes approximately fourteen pounds of food additives, 160 pounds of sugar and eight pounds of salt annually. Sugar consumption is a major concern.

Refined carbohydrates and sugar push your immune system down. Cell mediated immunity is depressed by 50% for 120 minutes after sugar indigestion. Sugar also competes with the absorption of Vitamin C into cells. A 100-gram portion of sugar can significantly reduce the capacity of white blood cells to engulf bacteria or cancer cells. Maximum immune suppression occurs one to two hours after ingestion and remains suppressed for up to five hours after feeding. Avoid sugar if you want a strong immune system.

Mineral and vitamin content in foods has dropped significantly due to soil depletion. The nutritional content in our foods have decreased because of soil depletion due to over production and addition of fertilizers, pesticides, fungal aids and monoculture. The CNN film series, *Toxic America*, notes that when America was discovered the top soil was 18-25". Today it is an average of 3-5 inches. Even when you eat fresh fruits and vegetables, the mineral and vitamin levels are so low, it seems prudent to supplement your diet with organic food concentrates.

The video points out that more people die each year of air pollution related illnesses such as asthma, respiratory allergies, lung and heart disease than automobile accidents. The series raises the alarm about the staggering levels of toxic chemicals dumped into our soil and waterways each year and comments that even the polar bears and the Inuit people in Greenland are now becoming toxic with the buildup of PCBs and DDEs in their bodies. The World Health organization estimates that "4.6 million people die each year from causes directly attributed to air pollution." (www.cnn.com/SPECIALS/2010/toxic.america/).

The Food and Drug Administration provides a list of the thousands of chemicals that are permitted into our foods in the United States (http://www.fda.gov/Food/IngredientsPackagingLabeling/FoodAdditivesIngredients/ucm091048.htm).

Also, the Toxic Release Inventory (TRI) Program tracks data related to toxic chemicals that may be harmful to the environment and human health. It is an Environmental Protection Agency Program (EPA) intended to inform the public as to what toxic chemicals are being released or being disposed of in communities in America. Information is self-reported by thousands of industries in the United States (http://www2.epa.gov/toxics-release-inventory-tri-program/2013-tri-national-analysis-introduction). The TRI annual report based on data reported by industries from the previous year are available to the public (http://www2.epa.gov/toxics-release-inventory-tri-program/tri-data-and-tools).

In the December 2013 Journal of Reproductive Toxicology, researchers Neltner, et al. reported that the US Food and Administration (FDA) allows "more than 10,000 chemicals...to be added, directly or indirectly, to human food" for purposes such as "preserving flavor, enhancing taste or appearance and to preventing spoilage". Legally food additives cannot be added to food unless they are deemed to be safe. The authors caution, however, that "80% of chemical additives directly—intentionally—added to food lack the relevant information needed to estimate the amount that consumers can safely eat" and that there are "data gaps in toxicity testing of chemicals allowed in food in the United States." (http://www.sciencedirect.com/science/article/pii/S0890623813003298).

In addition to making changes in your diet, you can decrease your exposure to toxins by substituting natural home and garden product options. A large selection of natural products are available in health food stores, super markets and on-line on sites such as mercola.com. Orange Guard, for example, is a natural broad range residual repellant and is safe to use around food, human and pets and as a weed killer you can use straight vinegar. We are not promoting any particular product; rather we are simply highlighting that there are many options available.

We recommend you download the questionnaire from the URL given below and fill it out to assess your risk of toxic exposure. There are questions related to lifestyle and various exposures that increase your risk to toxicity. We recommend that you fill it out before you start the cleanse and then again after.

Diet and Lifestyle

Symptoms of toxicity are often not well understood by the medical community.

In addition to environmental toxic exposure, we have internal exposure to toxins. Of concern are bleached and genetically modified grains, refined and artificial sugar, altered oils, Trans-fats, hydrogenate oils, artificial colors and other additives. In a sense our bodies have no idea what to do with these modified, processed foods. Soft drinks are also of concern. The active ingredients in soft drinks is phosphoric acid. Phosphoric acid leaches calcium from the bones and is a major contributing risk in osteoporosis. It can leach minerals at a high rate to alkalize acidity.

Our bodies need to try to break down and assimilate all the toxins that come from our diet. The Trans fats you consume will become embedded in the walls of your body rather than just passing through. So even with a 21-day detoxification program it will still take time to rid your body of not only the trans fats but also the accumulation of other toxins. It is best to avoid these over the long term and that is what the wellness solution is all about.

Weight gain, fatigue, headaches, allergies, joint and muscle pains, edema, anxiety, stress, hormonal function, skin rashes, sleep problems are all symptoms of toxic exposure. So, when we are looking at symptoms and how you feel, the question comes up, what effect does all this toxicity have on us? We see this in our practice all the time. Often it is misdiagnosed, not well understood by the medical community, but you take individuals who have weight gain issues, they go on diets but cannot lose weight. Sometimes that is a symptom of toxicity in the body resulting in chronic fatigue, headaches or allergies.

We have patients come to our office with year-round allergies. They are congested, have sinus problems, suffer from edema or joint aches and pains. Often it is a toxicity although it can be symptoms of other issues such as food allergies. We have to realize that these toxins affect everyone differently. It is important to pin point the possible causes of the symptoms as it can come from so many different things.

So again, the overwhelming idea with the wellness solution is to remove the toxicity, to give the body sufficient amount of proper nutrition supplemented by proper exercise to reduce stress. Often, you do not need to go chasing these symptoms that are creating these problems. If you just eliminate the bad stuff and add good stuff, then the symptoms may simply go away.

Toxins and free radicals can damage the energy producing powerhouse of the cells, the mitochondria leading to lower cellular function and fatigue. Toxins are poisons. Just like a hangover, toxins can trigger a number of symptoms including headaches, puffy eyes, face and swollen legs. Some cases of joint pain, anxiety disturbances PMS, chronic mucus production, recurrent infections, inability to concentrate, depression, mood changes, memory loss, sleep disturbances are associated with toxicity, leaky gut and bad diet. Unfortunately, our bodies were never meant to handle this level of exposure and our systems become overwhelmed.

The solution to pollution is dilution. As the toxic burden goes up the body must find more and more storage for these toxins and more fat or water weight is added to be used as toxic dump sites to protect the body from freely circulating toxins. Once created the body is very reluctant to get rid of the toxic dumps unless we first get rid of the toxins through a process of detoxification.

Detoxification: A 21-Day Purification Program

"If you can imagine, you can do it."
Walt Disney

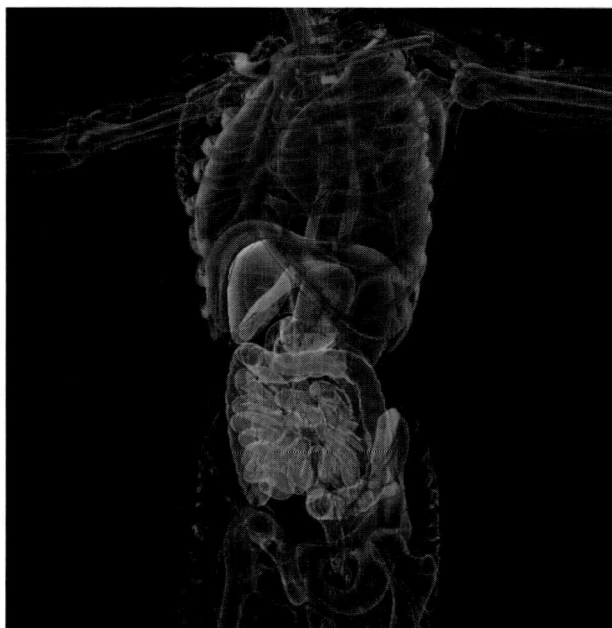

Detoxification Organs: Liver, Kidneys, Colon

Our bodies re wonderfully made and able to clear away toxins. So, let us look at how the body detoxifies, in particular how the intestinal track works. The food we eat must be properly digested. The lining in your gut should be tightly sealed to prevent leaky gut. Through a bad diet, constant use of nonsteroidal anti-inflammatory drugs (NSAID) or other causes, it becomes leaky. Higher amounts of harmful agents may be absorbed. This is known as leaky gut syndrome.

By completely dedicating yourself and by following all the guidelines of your recommended program, you are reaching out to tap into this powerful healing force within each one of us. Walt Disney said, "If you can imagine, you can do it." See yourself at the beginning of a new life, rich in health and learning. The body will follow.

The first phase of a cleanse is akin to getting your garbage packaged for pick up, while the second phase would be the actual garbage pickup, hopefully without spilling the garbage. There is no need to buy any products. We will be making some recommendations on supplements that can help the body eliminate the toxins quickly, different herbs, and different fibers. We will discuss different food groups, what to eat and what you should avoid and at what intervals you can introduce these different foods. We will also have a handout you can download that will summarize some of the things as well, something for you to reference back.

Do not cheat yourself out of the highest chance for the best possible outcome by eating non-approved foods. As your body starts to clean away food antigens from your blood stream as well as toxins that have been in storage, it now has the opportunity to seek out current health issues and resolve them.

Eating just a bite of food you are sensitive or allergic to can cause you to feel terrible as the body now has to deal with this acute reaction. Once your body becomes clearer you will become more sensitive to foods that are good for you. "You might never notice an empty can throw into the garbage, but you will always notice a gum wrapper on the golf course."

Frequency of urination may increase as the body is flushing out toxins. This is natural as the body starts to burn fat and normal insulin levels drop. This will level out after a few days. Increased bowel movements are also a natural response to increased clearing. Many today have forgotten what a complete bowel movement entails. Some people will experience a throbbing sensation in the head, generalized aches, itchy skin, or even a little fatigue. These symptoms are a normal response to clearing out poisons and should pass after the first day or so. Once you are past this you should start feeling better than you have in years. Hang in there.

The 21--Day Purification Program

"The natural healing force within each one of us is the greatest force in getting well."

Hippocrates

The 21-day purification program can also be called a detoxification. Hippocrates once said, "The natural healing force within each one of us is the greatest force in getting well." The 21-day detox program is just such an opportunity.

Days 1-10

Eat veggies only during the first ten days. Eat twice as many vegetables as fruit. Fifty per cent or more should be raw. If it is not raw, it should be slightly steamed or stir fried over low heat. Organic produce is recommended. Butter is excellent to use. Choose organic if possible. Avoid spreads, corn oil, vegetable oils, Crisco, safflower oil and all hydrogenated oils and Trans fats. This is vitally important to your success.

Drink at least eight to ten glasses of water each day. No caffeine, alcohol or tobacco. If you are a big coffee drinker and get a headache, brew a little bit of coffee and take a few sips to bring your headache down. Green tea is an excellent choice and while it has little caffeine it is acceptable during the program. Try new vegetables and fruit you have never tried before. Concentrate on high water, fiber vegetables for best results. Broccoli, cabbage, cauliflower, Brussel sprouts, leeks, bok choy. Remember no corn, white potatoes, and bananas, other than one half banana in a shake if desired.

Salad dressing is allowed but is very important you use only one of these, no exceptions, olive oil, and apple cider vinegar are good choices. Annie's brand specific approved balsamic vinaigrette.

Cilantro lime, French, green garlic, honey mustard, lemon olive raspberry, low fat roasted pepper vinaigrette, Tuscany Island. Please do not go beyond these parameters. Many dressings contain fructose, dairy, wheat. Good oils to use are coconut, red palm, olive, almond, sesame seed (cold expeller pressed only. Butter from organic, pasture-fed cows is best. Organic Agave nectar is fine. It only has 45 calories per tablespoon and a glycemic index of 14 and a glycemic load of 2.4. Xylitol has no calories and is from a natural source.

No beans, nuts, soy, corn, grains or dairy. After twenty-one days, they can be added back one at a time to evaluate food allergy reaction. No white potatoes, corn or grains of any kind. Sweet potatoes are recommended, but no more than one per day. Try adding butter and cinnamon.

Let us look briefly at nightshades and arthritis. Potatoes, tomatoes, hot peppers, eggplant, tamarins, pimentos, cayenne, Tabasco sauce are all classified as nightshade foods. People react to something called solanines in nightshade plants which can aggravate arthritis symptoms. So, if you happen to experience increased soreness and your arthritis symptoms acting up when you eat these list of plants, then it may be something you will want to avoid during the cleanse and long term if possible.

Days 11-21

After 10 days, you can add palm sized portions of fish back into your diet two to three times per day. Cold water ocean fish is the best. Choose wild Atlantic salmon, cod, etc. Avoid lake fish and farmed salmon as the fish can contain antibiotics, color and other additives. A little red organic meat, chicken or turkey every other day is acceptable. Eat only free-range, hormone and antibiotic free. Try sticking mostly with fish. Other than these additions do not add any other food back yet. Do not fry your food. Rather, lightly stir fry, steam, et cetera. Broiling, steaming, and roasting are also fine, but do not over-cook. Recommended foods to eat are steamed broccoli, brussels sprout, cabbage, kale, kohlrabi, mustard greens rutabaga and turnips. For deeper purification and increased weight loss and cancer fighting nutrients, concentrate on cruciferous vegetables like broccoli, cabbage, cauliflower, and brussels sprout. You should be feeling really good at this point. Congratulations so far.

That is basically it in a nutshell. The first ten days will see a lot of change, the next eleven days not so much. What most people notice if they have never done a cleanse before is that they are very toxic. The first three days can be a bit rough. With headaches, fatigue, or a bit of lightheadedness. That is normal as your body is trying to remove some of these toxins. After you have done several cleanses over a year or two, you might not notice much of a change which is a good thing. Make sure you stick to the foods and try not to deviate from that. You want to make sure you are drinking plenty of water, plenty of fluids and lots of tea and greens. That will help to eliminate lots of these toxins as well.

Remember to download the purification summary and the toxicity questionnaire from the links listed below. We also have a link to the purification kit from Standard Process that we have used. If you decide you want to use that, it gives you a protein shake, some extra fiber, green supplements. These are things that can help enhance the purification process. And make it a bit easier. It is kind of an all in one kit. You will still need to get all your fruits and vegetables and lean protein after day ten. But the nice thing about the kit is that it is all there and you are getting everything you need. So, we will make it available for you. We wish you the best of luck. If you have never done a cleanse before it is never too late to start. If you have done several in the past, we still recommend that you do one every six months or once a year.

Toxicity Questionnaire - http://thewellnesssolution.co/wp-content/uploads/2013/08/Toxicity_Questionnaire.pdf

Purification Summary - http://thewellnesssolution.co/wp-content/uploads/2016/01/Purification-Summary.pdf

Chapter 8

Clean Eating: Weight Loss and Vitality Through Healthy Eating

When you get good nutrients in your system, you change your physiology.

This chapter explores the eating well aspect of health and wellness. Although we have already touched on food, nutrition, supplementation and what a healthy diet looks like, this will provide a much deeper insight into the dimension of health. We discuss ways to help you to eat healthy every day, whether you are at home, at work or school, eating out, or on the road. We also present practical suggestions to encourage your kids to eat well.

Eating Clean

If you eat clean and exercise regularly your body will move towards the perfect equilibrium.

What does a good healthy diet look like? First and foremost, it has to be clean which means no processed or refined foods. Obviously, you will want to avoid chemicals, additives, artificial sweeteners and food colorings. The easiest way to do that is to eat food whole and organic whenever possible. Eat fresh fruits, vegetables, free-range meat, poultry and eggs, and avoid processed and refined products from boxes or bags. Eating clean is basically just that, eating food whole, the way it is meant to be eaten.

We have talked about this in the previous chapters, but we want to run the point home. A lot of us learn through repetition. We may have to hear the same or similar things several different times before it finally clicks home. You never make lasting meaningful change in your life until you own the why behind what you are doing. We are no different. We always need to be reminded of why we are doing what we are doing.

Be sufficient

Another component of a healthy diet is being sufficient. Obviously, you want to avoid things that make you toxic, while pursuing things in your diet that create sufficiency. Sufficiency is again is going to come through whole foods and the appropriate complement of those whole foods, such as meats, fruits and vegetables. You are going to want to have that good complement of micro nutrients, your vitamins, minerals, your phytonutrients which are going to be the right types of proteins, good healthy fats, good bulk forming fiber, and so on.

Again, you do not need to have a doctorate in nutrition to understand that. Eating healthy at the end of the day is simply eating whole foods that have always been around us. They are not coming out of a box or bag.

Also, we recommend some supplements you should be taking to avoid insufficiencies. Most of these concepts are fairly simple. It is easy to resort to fast foods and quick easy things we can eat, but they are not going to provide the nutrients we need. Many of these processed fast foods are fortified, but if you eat foods in their natural state, they should not need to be fortified. Try to eat foods that provide everything your body needs to have sufficient amounts of micro and macro nutrients for good health. These include proteins, healthy fats, healthy carbs, branch chain amino acids, vitamins, minerals, phytonutrients, omega-3 fatty acids, enzymes and fiber.

Avoid fad diets or diets that create deficiencies

A diet consisting of free range meats, fish, whole organic fruits and vegetables will provide most everything your body needs, while avoiding all the bad stuff. It is worth pointing out when you look at what the foundation of a good healthy diet entails. I dislike the word *diet* because many people associate the word diet with weight loss regimes when a diet is simply just what you eat on an ongoing basis. We recommend a good healthy diet for life.

We recommend avoiding the fad diets out there. Most of these diets can create deficiencies. You may lose some weight for the first couple of weeks but again the problem with that is that it is going to completely change your metabolism and in some ways, even shut it down. Often, your body is going to go searching for those calories elsewhere which is going to create abnormal cravings. It is hard to come out of that and expect to have a healthy, normal metabolism or normal appetite.

If your body is lacking certain nutrients, your body is going to have to slow down because your body is going to try to conserve the nutrients it has, so in the end you are going to lose out because as soon as you stop that diet you may balloon back to more than what you were when you started the diet. If you have some weight concerns and want to get the weight off a little bit quicker than by just eating cleanly, add an additional exercise component to your daily routine.

Basically, weight loss in a nutshell is simply consuming fewer calories than you need for your normal activities and then adding a bit of additional exercise as well to bring you to a kind of negative place for calories so your body will go after the fat for fuel. So, if you do that in a nice methodological process you are less likely to be hungry or have cravings. The weight will come off and that is dieting for weight loss in a nutshell. But again, in order to find a market, fad diet authors keep re-packaging their diets in different forms suggesting quick, miraculous weight loss results if people buy their book and follow their diet.

We recommend weight loss in a system, a program that is sustainable. Again, if you are eating something crazy like mostly grapefruit or carbohydrates or fats, these diets are not sustainable, so you have never learned to eat right for life. If you eat right, give your body what it needs and do not eat a lot of junk, your body is going to move to its ideal weight anyway. You do not need a short-term diet, just eat healthy and you will end up where you should be. And the weight can come off fairly quickly.

Two years ago, I had a patient who gave up all refined foods and ate mainly a lot of vegetables, fruit and meat. His weight steadily melted off. Within three months he dropped thirty pounds, ten pounds per month and he did it very healthfully. He was a big guy, so he ate a lot, but by substituting the junk food with whole healthy foods, he was able to lose weight without feeling hungry. He now feels great and his energy levels have never been better. For him there is no going back. I could not talk that guy out of this healthy diet because it is a diet he has now chosen for life. He hit this ideal weight and his body has stayed there. He is not counting any calories, he is not eating certain foods, he is not following any fads, he is just eating right and his body has come to that perfect equilibrium.

Supplementation to Optimize Health

Over farming has resulted in the depletion of nutrients in the soil. Often supplementation may be required for optimum wellness. It is not so much that we are just not eating the right foods, rather part of the problem is over farming. As a result, many of the nutrients in the soil have been depleted, consequently it is just more and more difficult to get that full complement of nutrients that we need. We recommend that eat the best you can and then supplement as needed. It is just like an insurance policy to make sure you are getting all the nutrients that you need.

Omega-3 fats for instance, may need to be supplemented because it is very difficult to eat enough good healthy, fatty fish, especially in states such as Colorado. In locations close to the ocean such as Seattle, you will probably have much more access to fish.

It is a similar situation for Vitamin D. For most of us who work indoors it is very difficult to get outside and get the appropriate amount of sun to produce a sufficient amount of Vitamin D. Additionally, people are concerned about the link between the sun and skin cancer, so without supplementation it may be difficult to get the needed Vitamin D.

If your diet does not include sufficient amounts of leafy green vegetables, such as collard greens, kale, lettuce and spinach or vegetables such as broccoli and cabbage, you may consider supplementing with Vitamin K which works as an adjunct to Vitamin D in maintaining bone health. It is also essential for blood clotting.

Probiotics, the beneficial bacteria may also need to be supplemented. Most of our food is quite sterile so we are not getting sufficient good bacteria necessary for optimum health. If you are already eating fermented foods, such as Kieffer, sauerkraut or Kimchi on a regular basis or drinking fermented tea such as Kombucha, additional probiotics may not be needed. If not, we recommend a probiotic which has a broad spectrum of healthy bacteria.

The accompanying Wellness Cookbook includes a number of great recipes if you choose to make your own fermented foods. You may also want to include a whole food multivitamin depending on your particular situation. Examine your diet and determine what areas can be beefed up a bit with additional supplementation.

Eating Well While You Are Out and About

How do you eat well while eating out? The first place to start is to ask yourself how much are you eating out and why. Generally, it is difficult to eat well while you are eating out. In most restaurants, particularly in fast food restaurants most foods are going to be to be processed, refined and have lots of sodium, so the best things you can do is to limit eating out.

Put some forethought into what does your schedule look like during any given week. There are a number of things you can do if you plan ahead to ensure that you are eating healthier, whether you are at work, on the road, or just out and about. We tend to cook well when eating at home, but when eating out it is hard to emulate that, so what we tend to do is to cook a lot more for dinner and package that up in some glassware and take it work the next day, so then we can at least emulate what we are eating at home while we are at work.

But what do you do about situations such as the weekends while you are grocery shopping or out with the family and things are running late? The kids are hungry and are pressuring you to go to eat somewhere, so in that situation you may end up going to a fast food or chain restaurant. What restaurant, of course, depends on the area you are in and what restaurants are available. Assuming there are some options, think about the healthy foods you are eating at home and what restaurant can provide the most nutritious option. Where can you get healthy meats, fruits, vegetables, whole grain breads, foods that are not deep fried stuff or with a lot of added chemicals.

Check out restaurant menus in advance. It is going to take a bit of work, but you can save time by checking the menus and reviews on line. What restaurants would you go to if you are looking for that? When you choose a restaurant, do not be afraid to ask the waiter or waitress to make some changes or to do something special.

If you go to a restaurant and want a cob salad for example, you can ask to have the heavy ranch type dressing substituted for a bit of squeezed lemon or some balsamic vinegar. If there is breaded chicken on your salad, ask what it would take to get grilled chicken instead. There is probably something on the menu that has grilled chicken and most restaurants can just grab that and put it on the salad instead. So, do not be afraid to ask for things like that. It is a simple request and most waiters or waitresses will accommodate.

When our family goes to a Tex Mex type of place like Chipotle, there are often options for whole fresh ingredients, tomatoes, lettuce, guacamole, which is basically avocados with spices added in and different types of salsa with fresh tomatoes in it, so it is pretty easy to pick out something that has the different food groups you need and have them put it into a burrito bowl. A lot of places have grilled chicken salads where you can easily substitute a few things to make a healthy meal. If you choose to have an Asian dish such as a stir fries, you will want to watch the sauces. Teriyaki has a lot of sugar, soy sauce contains genetically modified ingredients, and the Asian meal may also have MSG. In a pinch, however, an Asian stir fry can really work.

When travelling, you can go to the grocery store and get some fresh items and make a quick lunch instead of stopping at a fast food restaurant. We often pick up healthy items in grocery stores, for example, you can buy some turkey meat, put it on to some leaf lettuce, add some other vegetables with a bit of spicy mustard, roll it up into an appetizing leaf lettuce sandwich. We do that almost every time we are out of town. It is simple to go to the grocery store the night before and grab some food for the next day or two.

So, a lot of this is just planning ahead, where you are going and what is along the way. You may want to grab a cooler to keep foods fresh during your travels. Most hotel rooms will have a fridge and if nothing else, they will have an ice machine, so you can replenish the ice in your cooler. We frequently go to Denver with our family and we always take a cooler now so that we can grab healthy foods along the way and keep them fresh. Without the cooler, you may be tempted to stop at a drive through fast food restaurant instead of eating something healthy, consequently jeopardizing your diet.

To summarize, avoid fast food restaurants as much as possible. Look for lean meats, fruits, vegetables. Burrito bowls at

Chipotles consisting of meat, grilled veggies, salsa, guacamole, lots of green vegetables are an option, but avoid the sour cream, cheese and rice. Grilled chicken salads are another healthier choice, but avoid creamy dressing, croutons and cheese. Use freshly squeezed lemon or balsamic vinegar and olive oil makes a very healthy dressing. Asian stir fry with lean meats, lots of fresh veggies but avoid sugary sauces and rice or have some brown rice sparingly. Avoid MSG and GMO soy sauce.

On the road, opt for grocery store lunch. Thin slices of turkey breasts wrapped in leaf lettuce with avocado and an organic apple are healthy choices. Again, it is probably not going to be completely organic, free range and all those things, but in a pinch, it can be a reasonably healthy option. So often there are some good choices there.

There are now a few chain restaurants offering options with natural ingredients. Chipotle Mexican Grill and Panera are two examples. Neither restaurant now uses any antibiotics or other drugs in their meat or poultry. Burger King no longer uses antibiotics for growth promotion, but it does use antibiotics for disease prevention (http://www.greenerchoices.org/products.cfm? product=animalag1115&pcat=food; GreenerChoices.org/animalag; www.ConsumerReports.org., Jan. 2016). In Canada, the A & W hamburger chain has stopped using hormones, steroids, antibiotics or preservatives in their beef and chicken (http://www.newswire.ca /news-releases/aw-canada-is-canadas-first-national-burger-estau rant-to-serve-better-beef-raised-without-added-steroids-or-hor mones-512988831.html).

As consumers become more vocal in demanding healthier food options, restaurants and supermarkets are going to provide increasingly greater options of healthier and organic foods.

Clean out your body and your body will actually start to crave good things.

Getting Your Kids to Eat Well

Getting your kids to eat well is sometimes easier said than done. With hectic weekly schedules, soccer, gymnastics, choir, and so on, with deceptive marketing of unhealthy foods to kids, the practice of rewarding kids with candies and other unhealthy junk, it is not an easy task to convince your kids to eat healthy. What happens when your kids want to eat only chicken nuggets dipped in plum sauce and drink soda, how do you approach that?

Again, if we can go back to the concept, clean out your body and your body will actually start to crave good things, but how do you go about doing that, especially when it comes to kids? As a starter, get the junk out of the house, the soda, candy, sugary cereals, sugar-laden yogurts, and so on. Clean out the fridge and cupboards and replace the bad stuff with good stuff. Bring out the fresh fruit and keep it out and available. Get rid of the high fructose corn syrup products, items with artificial sweeteners, hydrogenated oils, dyes, processed and refined foods, meats and chicken injected with antibiotics, hormones or fillers, canned goods and water containers with BPA. These are all harmful to everyone, but particularly to children with developing bodies. This may seem like an overwhelming task, but it is not that difficult. Most kids will eat lean protein such as chicken breasts, turkey, eggs, steak and lean ground beef. If you end up buying processed luncheon meats, make sure that they are nitrate or nitrite free. Make the food fun by cutting into small pieces or shapes. Consider a children's multivitamin, omega-3 fish oil and vitamin D supplement.

Start by having a conversation with your children about eating healthy. Discuss what it means to eat right and why important in order for their brains and bodies to work better. Most kids are pretty sharp and they will pick up on what you are trying to say. If they understand the why of what you are trying to do, they are not going to rebel against it as much. At the same time, you do not want to take everything away and be food tyrant at home. They will rebel against that.

As you work towards changes towards a healthier diet for the kids, it may be helpful to make some concessions. You may permit them to have one soda per week, such as a Mexican coke which contains cane sugar rather than high fructose corn syrup. Once the kids are old enough to make decisions on their own they may decide to completely eliminate the soda. Even if you permit periodic less healthy items, but that at the same time clear out much of the junk food, you have come a long way.

One of the most important changes to make is to supplement the children's diet with nutritious foods so that you can negotiate with your kids to eat the healthy stuff and then maybe they can have something not as healthy afterwards. After they eat all the healthy stuff they will not be as hungry and are less likely to crave the junk. It would be a challenge to attempt to eliminate all the bad stuff all at once. It is better to add good stuff and watch the bad stuff go away. Just leave the bad stuff out and it will be just a natural progression. For kids start with them slowly introducing a few good things initially and at the same time have a conversation about limiting or eliminating some bad things. Most families should be able to do that quite easily. Over a period of a month or two, start eliminating certain things and then over time the kids are not going to notice the bad stuff is gone.

There are many simple additional ways to get your kids to eat healthy and to start to crave healthy foods rather less junk foods. Have a fresh fruit bowl within easy reach. Provide healthy snacks, fresh whole organic fruit sliced up and ready to eat, a bowl of mixed raw organic almonds, cashews and walnuts, cut up carrots, celery, small bits of organic dark chocolate, treats such as freeze dried vegetable and fruit snacks and desserts, such as our lentil bars and coconut oil snacks (see recipes in the accompanying Wellness cookbook). Some children like to dip their vegetables in almond butter which is a healthy alternative to peanut butter, so you may want to have that available.

Instead of serving processed chicken nuggets, grill some chicken and cut it into small pieces. Serve it with a healthy dip. Kids often enjoy poultry and meats cut into small pieces and dipping the pieces into a sauce. Another suggestion would be having your kids make their own taco salads. Kids enjoy adding all the different toppings to their personalized taco. Replace the bad things and put in the good thigs, and in time your children will begin to prefer healthy food over junk food.

We recommend you consider some type of supplementation for kids. Maybe a children's multivitamin especially if they are not eating that well, but make sure it is a whole food multivitamin. You do not want to give a developing child synthetic vitamins. The omega 3 fish oil is very important. Many parents assume that omega 3 is only important for adults, but children with developing brains need those nutrients just as much if they are not big fish eaters, which unfortunately encompasses most children.

Also, vitamin D3 supplements are something to be considered as well. A lot of kids are not getting outside enough to get a sufficient amount of the sunshine vitamin in order to build healthy bones. Rather, they spend most of their time indoors, at school or inside on their iPods or playing video games, and that is a whole other conversation, so if that is the situation with your children, make sure they have adequate supplementation such as a multivitamin, probiotic, omega 3 oil or vitamin D, if needed. Alternatively, there are a number of other ways to ensure that sufficient nutrients are incorporated into your child's diet such as freshly juiced green drinks and other nutritious shakes. So, decide what your children may be lacking and supplement the deficiencies accordingly.

Some healthy recipes can be found in our cookbook in paperback at https://www.amazon.com/dp/B01LK2VBA4. As a gift for purchasing this book, you can also download your free copy at http://thewellnesssolution.co/freebook/

Chapter 9

Exercise for Wellness: Fun and Enjoyable Exercises for Optimal Health

WITH THE MYRIAD OF CONFLICTING ADVICE, HOW DO WE DECIDE WHAT EXERCISES ARE APPROPRIATE FOR OUR PARTICULAR BODY AND LIFESTYLE?

This chapter focuses on exercise for optimal wellness. In the third chapter, *Exercise and Nutrition for Optimal Health*, we gave you a simple starter program, however, in this chapter we are taking it another step up by delving a bit deeper into weight bearing exercises. We will discuss what is meant by fitness and look at the difference between cardio and weight training types of exercises. We will explore the types of exercises you need to be doing to meet your particular needs.

Exercise is undoubtedly a crucial component of a healthy lifestyle, but where does one start? There can be a lot of confusion there. We see people in the gym all the time doing all kinds of different sort of stuff that could be doing more harm than good. We will shed some more light on that in our exercise handouts and videos.

We have put together a clear-cut research-based overview of exercises our bodies were designed for, specifically, the types of exercises you need to be doing to meet the needs of your particular body and lifestyle. We will discuss resistance type of exercises, cardio and weight training. We have included full length functional movement exercise videos created exclusively for the Wellness

Solution series. as well as a series of body weight workouts that you will be able to stream right from your computer.

We will also share an interesting, rather different alternative type of exercise program for those with limited time on their hands.

What is Fitness?

EVERYONE SEEMS TO HAVE THEIR OWN DEFINITION OF FITNESS

In our search for a definition of fitness, we found that there were not many good ones. Rather, there were numerous similar, rather simplistic definitions of fitness. The Oxford English Dictionary, The Merriam-Webster, The American Heritage and the Free Dictionary similarly define fitness as "the quality, condition or state of being physically fit, healthy or strong" (http://www.oed.com/; http://www.merriam-webster.com/dic tionary/fitness; https://ahdictionary.com/; http://www.thefreedic tionary.com/fitness). Your Dictionary states fitness is "being in good physical shape or being suitable for a specific task or purpose" (http://www.yourdictionary.com/fitness).

None of the definitions are particularly helpful in shedding clarity as to what fitness actually means to a particular individual. Additionally, there are a myriad of other definitions put forth by experts and lay people alike. Everyone seems to have their own version of what it means to be fit.

However, after looking at numerous definitions of fitness, we came across a definition by Doug McGuff and John Little that we like: "a bodily state of being physiologically capable of handling challenges that exist above a resting threshold of activity." In this book, we have talked a lot about the concepts of adaptability, whether it is adaptability with your emotional health, whether it is adaptability with your physiology or the structure of your body or your muscles. So, we really like this definition because it gets to the key point that your level of fitness is how adaptable you are to a certain amount of stress or environmental changes that come your way. If you cannot adapt to something, you end up succumbing to it and its stressors. So, we do like this definition.

In the past, we never thought about trying to define what fitness is. We just assumed we knew what fitness was until we tried to define it. Things change depending on the particular fitness level we are currently in, so for a marathon runner it is going to be completely different than for a someone who sits at a desk all day. It is completely dependent on what their activities are. When you are thinking about wanting to be in a good state of fitness, then the question is what should a typical person's state of fitness be. Again, it depends on what kind of activities they are looking for. If someone wants to go from a couch potato just to a better state of fitness and they have no intention of running a marathon or climbing Mount Everest, what should that look like?

With the Wellness Solution, we endeavor to answer that question as to what that should that look like. A better state of fitness that creates healthier physiology in the body, gives you more energy, more adaptability and so forth. With some of these weight bearing, body weight exercises accompanying this chapter, we think we can get to that place.

Cardio or weights?

DO RUNNING MARATHONS OR PUMPING WEIGHTS TO BUILD LARGE MUSCLES EQUATE WITH BETTER HEALTH?

So then again, is cardio good for us? Let us expand on that. A lot of people think that individuals going to the gym doing all these exercises must be very healthy. We see people in the gym all the time doing all kinds of different stuff, but at times they can simply be hurting themselves if the exercises are not done properly. Lifting weights can cause injury if not done properly or if the body is unable to adapt and appropriately tolerate the weight. When you look at some of these individuals down the road, they may have heart damage, arthritis or have other problems that have come about because they are doing way too much for what the body was designed for. They may have wear and tear on their joints, and if their diet is not healthy, they may also have excessive inflammation which can cause further degradation of the cartridges and the joints.

So, it is a bigger picture than simply working out at a gym. Simply going to the gym does not necessarily equate with better health in the long term. People need to step back a bit and decide what they want, whether they want to simply just look good or be healthy as well because there is a big difference. A muscle-bound person is not necessarily fit, and similarly, someone who can run hundred miles is not necessarily healthy. So what type of exercise should you be doing, cardio or resistance type of weight training exercises or both? There can be a lot of confusion there. We have observed in our practices individuals following fitness trends that look pretty good but end up getting over trained because they fail to allow their bodies enough recovery time. They lose their form and they end up getting sick. We see trends like this happening particularly after a lot of lifting.

This can be a concerning issue especially when you consider the fact that the human structure has to have time to adapt. When the body is stressed by wear and tear on the muscles and injury, it takes time to heal and adapt properly. If you are exerting your body to an increasing intensity, you need enough time for your body to build collagen. The tendons and muscles need to be sufficiently strong to be able to sustain the exercises again. When you are pushing yourself to the absolute maximum at any point, whether it is pushing weights to build muscles and strength or engaging in long sustained running, it is going to create a lot of wear and tear and not stimulate the necessary hormone production.

What was the human body really designed for? We suggest a balance between cardio and weights. Simply by just doing weights or by running you are going to stimulate your cardio system and your muscles, so you cannot separate one from the other. If you look at our ancestors, they were not running marathons. They would typically have short bursts of high intense activity, but they were not running any marathon. At the same time, they were not lifting weights to build large muscles either. What they experienced was a balance between high intensity and short duration exercise.

There is a lot of research in support of high intensity shorter duration interval training as being more in tune with what our bodies were designed for. Shorter intensity and shorter duration exercises may be a healthier option for the body and cardiovascular system than long sustained duration of running or cycling or whatever so that the body is adequately stimulated without causing a lot of wear and tear.

Body Weight Exercises

THE ADVANTAGE OF BODY WEIGHT EXERCISES IS THAT YOU CAN SIMPLY USE YOUR OWN BODY WEIGHT FOR THE EXERCISES.

In this chapter, we will jump right in and present a great program of body weight exercises. These exercises are probably a bit more intense than the ones we introduced in the third chapter, *Nutrition and Exercise Fundamentals*, but we wanted to make sure you were doing at least some exercises earlier in the Wellness

Solution series. For those of you who may have just got off the couch and have not been that conditioned or have not done much in a while, these exercises are a good place to start. Any of these exercises can be done at your own level of fitness depending where you are at.

So, if you have been doing the exercises presented earlier all along or have already come to the Wellness Solution with a fairly good level of fitness, you can take these exercise to the next level. You can simply increase or decrease the intensity depending where you are currently at. The nice thing about body weight type exercises is that you do not need any machines or weights. You can, however, incorporate dumbbells, kettlebells or a medicine ball, but they are not essential as simply using your own body weight will suffice. It is all fairly low tech. Like with any exercise, make sure to do a warm up.

We have a series of six body weight based exercise videos that you can stream to your computer or mobile device. These videos incorporate movements that stimulate a lot of different muscles and joints. The videos are accompanied by a handout that explains what you will be doing and the number of repetitions of each exercise. Make sure to print out and follow the instructions in the handout. The first video is a warm up video; the second demonstrates jumps and lunges, great functional movements; the third video looks at push-ups and dumbbells; and the fourth video shows squats jumps, along with kettlebells. If you have never worked with kettlebells before, you may find them fun to use. On the other hand, if kettlebells are not for you, the exercises can be done without them. Video five illustrates sumo squats and video six focuses on more mat work.

For those of you who are time conscious but still want to get some exercises during the week, we present an interesting alternative in the next chapter.

Exercise Videos

You can download an outline of all the exercises here http://thewellnesssolution.co/wp-content/uploads/2012/02/Exercise-Outline.pdf

The Warm Up Video: http://youtu.be/smlMfEkZmPM.

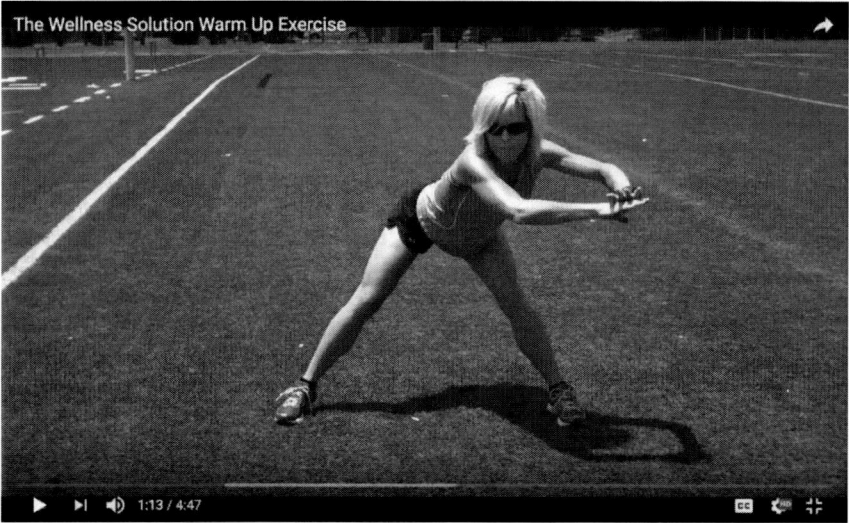

Jumps and Lunges video: http://youtu.be/w2xliLwdm_k

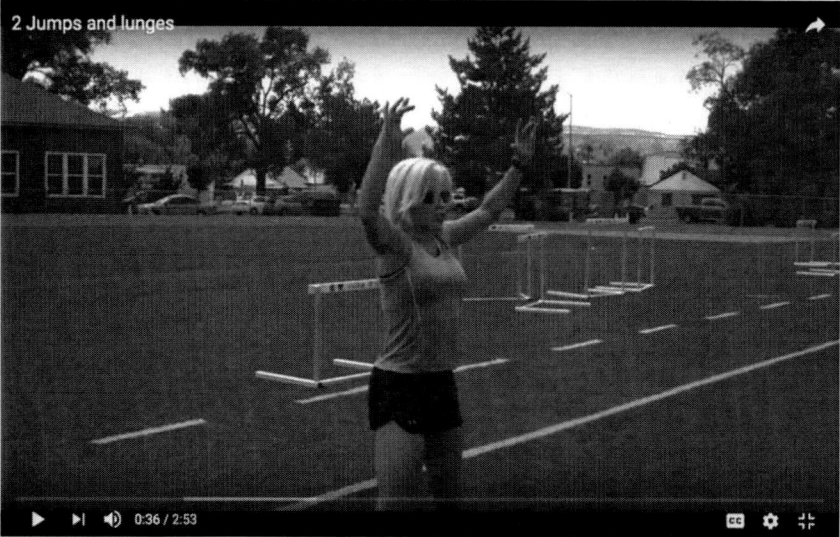

Dumbells and Pushups video: http://youtu.be/4zNMA8iGIXw

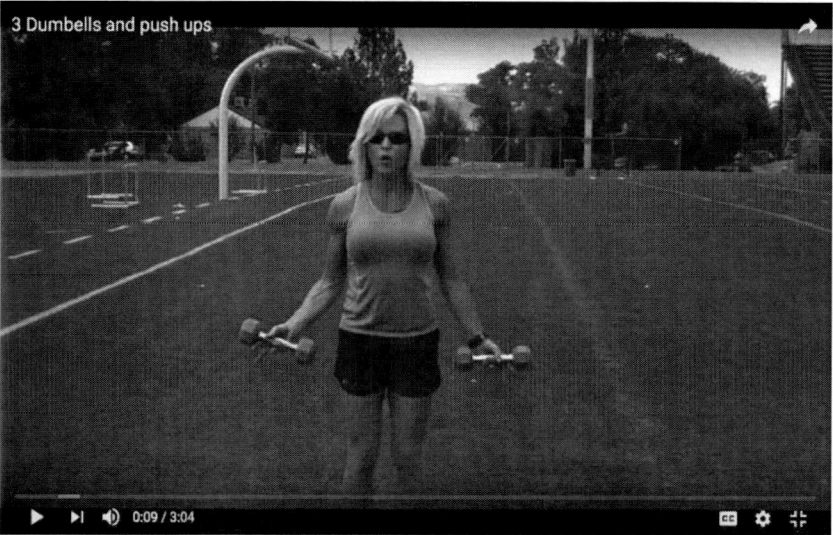

Kettle Bell and Squat Jumps Video:
http://youtu.be/G2dVQIyoxM4

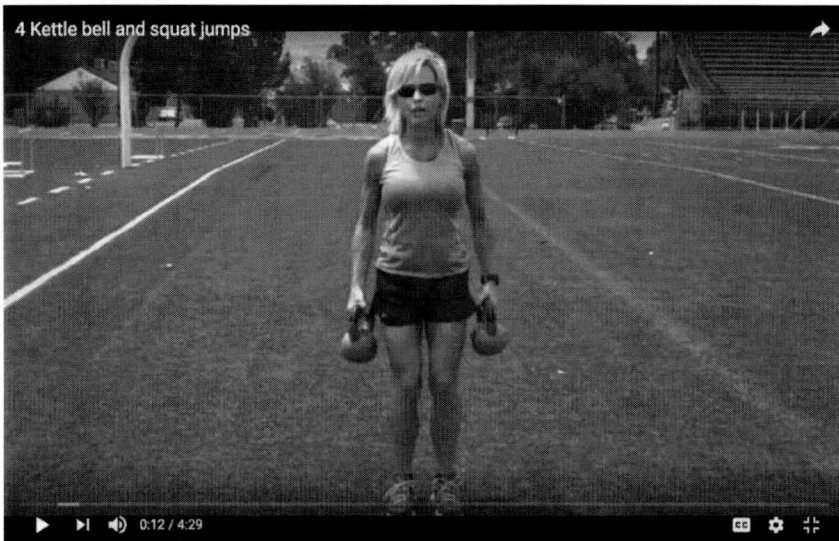

Sumo Squats Video: http://youtu.be/688yWDoJnqg

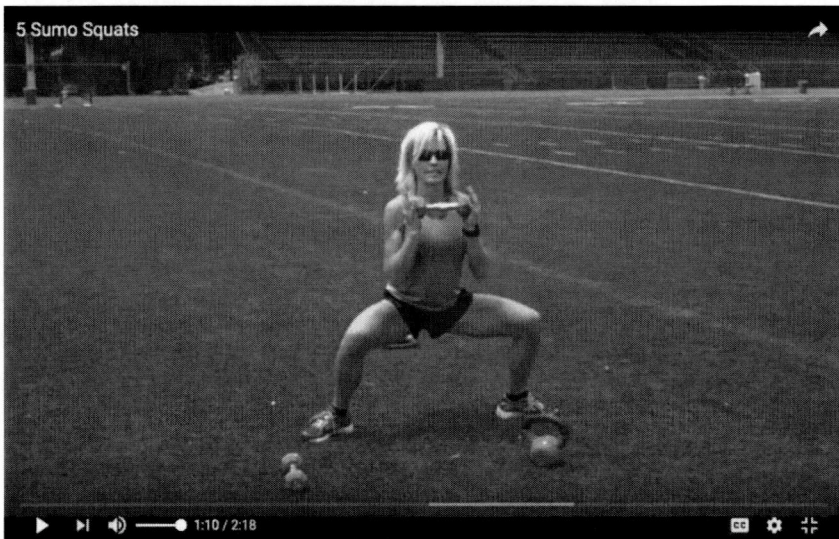

Mat Work Video: http://youtu.be/b2V9sPzI94k

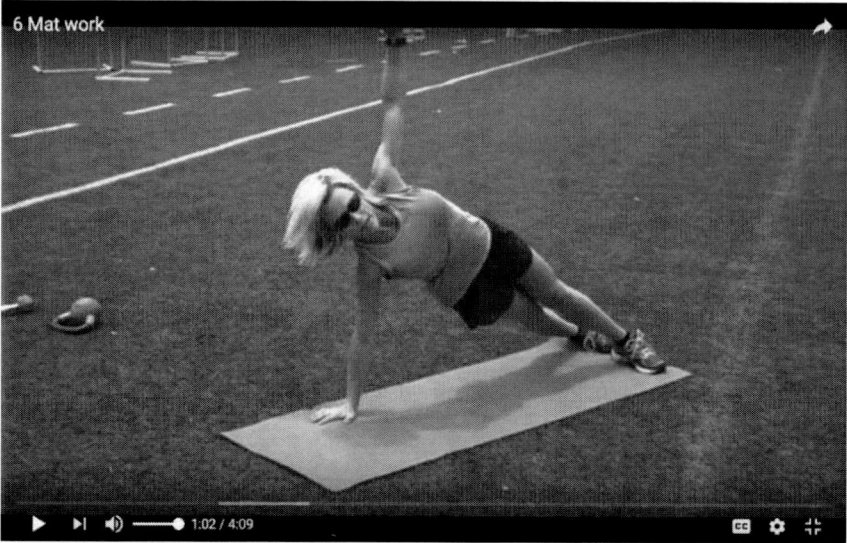

Alternatives for Those with Limited Time

John Little and Doug McGuff, in *Body by* Science (available on Amazon.com), present a very different alternative exercise program to meet the needs of individuals with limited time on their hands. They offer primarily a strength and body building program which requires only twelve minutes per week. Although it is somewhat controversial and obviously not for everyone, we have decided to mention the program because it does present a different option for those individuals pressed for time. Again, you cannot do this workout program if you are wanting to train for a marathon since you have to do the running and put in the miles, or if you are a tennis player you cannot expect to become a pro tennis player if you do not spend the time doing the necessary training.

This program entails basically five different exercises you do until you are maxed out. They are: rows with hands vertical; chest press; pull downs; shoulder press; and leg press. The exercises should be started at eighty per cent of a one repetition maximum or for about ninety seconds until you cannot do any more. You work on one set of each exercise for approximately ninety seconds each. The authors postulate that with these high intensity exercises, you will be stimulating different parts pf your body that can help build muscle and increase fat stimulation and cardio function.

The authors stress that these exercises should be done no more than once per week because it is going to take seven to ten days for your body to recover. They note that people trying to exercise to that level in a shorter amount of time will get weaker because their body hasn't recovered enough. As we mentioned, it is not for everyone, but it is an alternative for someone who does not have a lot of time and wants to improve their underlying fitness and cardiovascular system without putting in hours and hours in the gym.

Make sure you view the exercise videos. Definitely get in there and try out the program.

Chapter 10

Mind Body Healing: How to Create Optimal Health Using Your Thoughts

Stress and the Mind Body Connection

Extended periods of stress can have a profound impact on the body's ability to fend off disease and sickness.

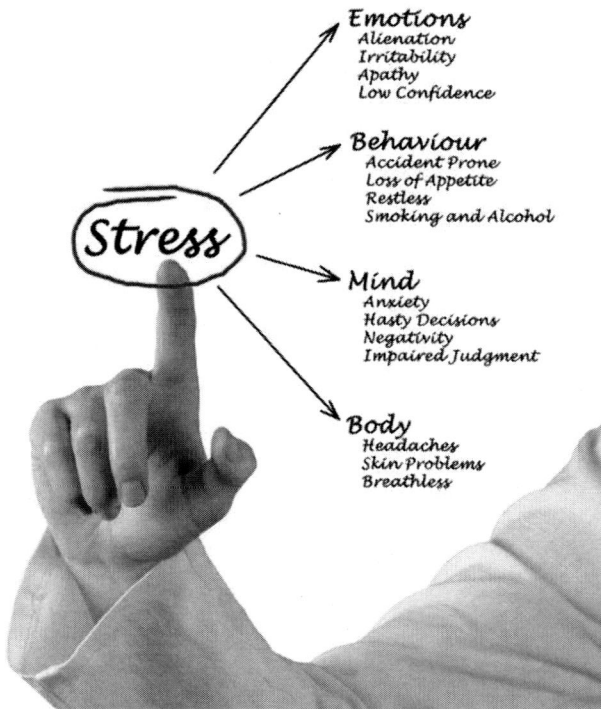

In this chapter, we explore the mind-body connection to give you a deeper appreciation for this interconnection. We live our lives in three dimensions, physical, biochemical and emotional. Though our bodies are designed to adapt to the environment, too much stress for too long in any of these dimensions can have detrimental repercussions on physical health. In this chapter, we present some simple and highly effective strategies to reduce and even eliminate stress in the three dimensions to reduce the possible negative toll on our overall physical health. Though our bodies are designed to adapt to the environment, too much stress for too long in any of these dimensions is the root cause of all disease and sickness, whether it be Type 2 diabetes from prolonged elevated sugar, degenerative spinal disease from poor posture or inflammation or ulcers from unresolved stress.

We are always going to attempt to counter our stressors. Our body has the ability to be able to adapt to those stressors whether it is physical impacts on our body, particular types of foods, or challenging emotional situations. Our bodies have the ability to adapt to those stressors up to a point, but when it cannot adapt, that is when our body starts to break down and that failure to adapt can eventually turn into diseases. It is a matter of balancing the positive stressors in all three categories with the negative ones. The more positive the stressors, the healthier you are going to end up being. and the more negative the stressors, the more compromised your health will become.

Physical stressors

Physical stressors create positive or negative physiological changes depending on your body's ability to adapt effectively to the intensity of the impact.

When we talk about stress what we typically think of is emotional stress, rather than physical stress. Physical stressors can be equally concerning as they influence the body both externally and internally, thereby contributing to physiological changes.

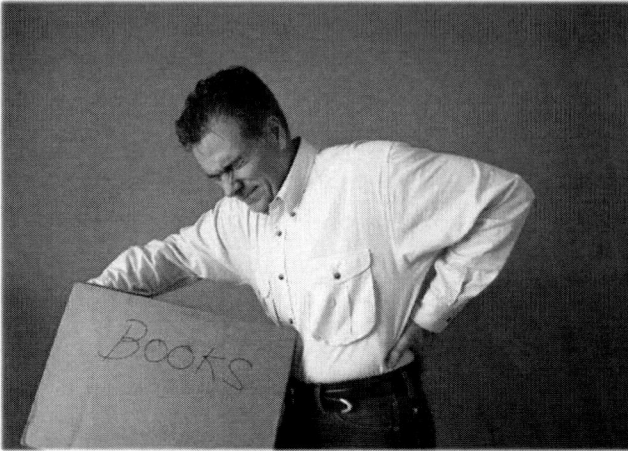

Examples of negative physical stressors would be poor posture, injuries, sprains and strains. Slouching forward can result in pain on your ligaments and muscles. Over time the body may not be able to compensate for the stress caused by the bad posture resulting in damage, possibly chronic. Negative physical stressors such as spring strain injuries and whiplash type of injury are often caused by car accidents. The force is simply too intense for the body to be able to adapt. These examples of physical stressors are considered negative stressors because we simply cannot adapt to them.

On the other hand, physical stressors can also be positive. They include any activity that creates forces on the body that trigger a positive physiological change.

Positive physical stressors would be stretching and other types of exercises. However, positive stressors like exercise and stretching can also be negative if you do too much and overwhelm your body's ability to adapt. For example, if you run a marathon and are not trained properly that could turn out to be a negative physical stress. It is important to look into the context of your exercise routine to ensure that you give yourself sufficient recovery time between exercise sessions so that your body can heal and adapt. That is something we often do not think about. When you put a physical stressor into the body it is going to take a while for your body to adapt and to create the change and when you counter that stress again next time you can do better. That is what exercise is intended for.

Biochemical stressors

Practically every medication encompasses some sort of chemical that creates some sort of change or physiological shift or side effect in the body.

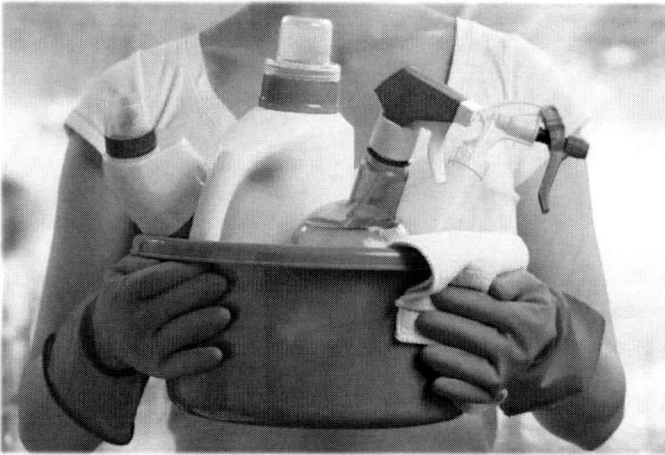

Biochemical stressors also create a positive or negative change or physiological shift in the body. Negative biochemical stressors include food additives, refined sugar, refined carbohydrates, environmental toxins, cleaning supplies, pollution and medications.

Practically every medication encompasses some sort of chemical that creates some sort of change or physiological shift or side effect in the body. Sometimes the symptom the medication is designed to treat is less problematic than the resulting side effects created by the medication.

On the other hand, positive biochemical stressors create desirable physiological shifts in your body. They include such things as having an appropriate diet that includes an adequate consumption of dietary fiber, vegetables and fruits and other roughage with different micronutrients that break down in the body to enhance the digestive process.

Emotional stressors

The inability of our brain to adapt to certain circumstances, real or imaginary has direct impact on the physiology of our body.

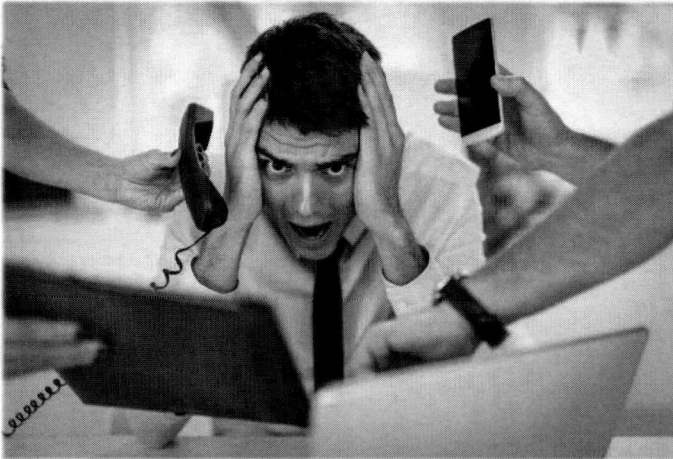

Like physical and biochemical stressors, emotional stressors can be positive or negative. Positive emotional stressors would be such things as laughing or crying. The emotional stressors release endorphins that come from those experiences.

Negative stressors are the result of an inability to adapt to various circumstances that we encounter in our daily lives. Negative emotional stressors include such things as fear, anger, pain or resentment. A number of research studies have concluded emotional stressors at the particular moment changes your physiology, the makeup of what's happening in your blood stream. So, imagine if you are in a state of resentment or anger, frustration or anxiety for weeks or months or years at a time, it can absolutely have a negative impact on your health. Although emotional stress is something that happens in your mind, it changes the physiology in your body.

This is nothing to be taken lightly. The inability of our brain to adapt to certain circumstances, real or imaginary has direct impact on the physiology of our body. We often have choices as to how to deal with the circumstances we encounter in our environment. You can choose to interpret many of these negative stressors you encounter as good or bad or in whatever way you like. A fear situation such as talking in public, for example, for someone that may cause a significant negative stress, while for someone else it might not be an issue. You have the choice to deal with the emotional stressor in a positive, negative or in a neutral manner. There are techniques to help you to change a negative stress into a positive one.

Three Secrets to Stress Management

Though our bodies are designed to adapt to the environment, too much stress for too long in any one of the three dimensions can result in disease and sickness.

We will present three simple, effective strategies to reduce or even eliminate stress in the three mind-body connecting areas.

As mentioned previously, we live our lives in three dimensions: physical, biochemical and emotional. The three dimensions are interconnected. Stress in any one of these dimensions will have an impact on the other. Though our bodies are designed to adapt to the environment, too much stress for too long in any of these dimensions can result in disease and sickness. Stress in the emotional dimension can affects our physical and biochemical health. The most effective strategy to manage physical stress is consistent exercise and stretching, activities that stimulate the body in a physical manner.

Biochemical stress is best countered by eating clean whole, organic foods. Avoid processed junk food and food additives. Avoid prescription medication if at all possible. Also, take high quality whole food multivitamins, omega 3 fish oil, vitamin D3, and a probiotic. Your body can adapt to that for a while but eventually it is going to be a problem. Providing all the nutrients the body needs to heal, adapt and function right are crucial for countering biochemical stressors.

Effective emotional stress management includes a daily routine of strategies such as daily positive affirmations, prayer and meditation. In addition to helping you to simply feel calm and relaxed, these techniques will help to decrease the alpha sympathetic nervous system to allow for the relaxation of the arteries and to decrease high blood pressure. These techniques will positively change your physiology.

First thing in the morning before you go to work, go through some positive affirmations. Instead of thinking about how poor your life is or the things you do not like in your life, think about, visually think about some of the positive things in your life or positive things you would like to come into your life. Verbalize that in a present day tense as well. Everyone can think of good things in their lives even when you have a habit of focusing on the negative. Get in the habit of thinking about the positive things in your life. This will not only change your mindset, but it will attract more positive energy and more positive people to you. It is magnetic, kind of like a law of attraction. You see some people who are always doom and gloom. It seems like bad things always happen to them. They will get into three car accidents in the same year. What is going on there? They appear to be attracting negatives into their lives.

Six Steps to Elicit the Relaxation Response

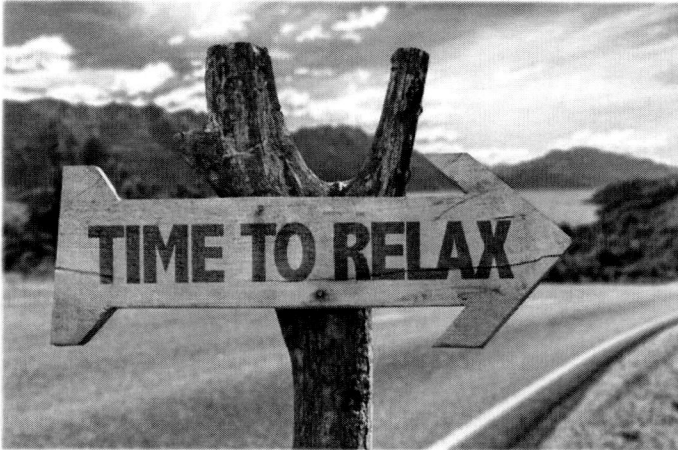

Dr. Herbert Benson, founder pf the Mind/Body Medical Institute in Massachusetts (http://www.relaxationresponse.org/) formulated stress management techniques popularized in his book, *The Relaxation Response* (https://www.amazon.com/Relaxation-Response-Herbert-Benson/dp/0380006766).

Benson's *Relaxation Response* was original inspired by the research he did looking at patients with high blood pressure (hypertension). He had his patients do this particular technique once a day for 20 minutes. He found that simply by having his patients follow this technique, he was able to get their blood pressure down significantly and in many cases permanently.

The following is an excerpt of Benson's stress management technique reprinted with permission from Dr. Benson's book, the Relaxation Response (pp. 162-163):

- Sit quietly in a comfortable position
- Close your eyes
- Relax all your muscles, beginning at your feet and progressing up to your face. Keep them relaxed.

You can use it at any time of the day. Find a quiet, comfortable place where you can relax in a chair, close your eyes and relax your muscles. You can do the exercises progressively. Begin with your feet and move up to your face and head. You could also do the exercises at night to help you to relax and fall asleep. This technique is particularly helpful if your mind is racing and you need to get out of that.

The biggest part of trying to create that relaxation response is the breathing. So, what you want to do is to breath very slowly through your nose and then try to breath even more slowly back out through your mouth. So, if it takes you four seconds to breath in, try to take eight seconds to breath out. Each time you do that try to make it go slower and slower to the point where you are only taking a breath maybe once or twice a minute. This is a highly effective exercise to help you to switch out of that fight or flight portion of your nervous system and get you to start relaxing. You can continue that for approximately ten to twenty minutes

Become aware of your breathing. As you breathe in, say the word "one" silently to yourself. Do the same as you breath out. Breathe easily and naturally.

Continue for ten to twenty minutes. You may open your eyes to check the time, but do not use an alarm. When you finish sit quietly for several minutes, at first with your eyes closed and later with your eyes open. Do not stand up for a few minutes. You can do some visualization while you do this as well. Think of yourself on a quiet beach somewhere. Appropriate breathing is a key component of this technique.

Breathe slowly into your nose and even more slowly out. The most important thing is not to get stressed out whether you are doing this right. So, just relax into it and you might notice as you go along from day to day that you get a bit better with the technique and you find yourself getting into a relaxation response a bit more quickly. Just pace yourself and go with it. We have provided you with a link to a handout that you can download to use as a reference. After a few times, you will not need to look at the handout anymore.

With practice, you will find it easier and easier to clear your mind. For some of you, it will be difficult at first and perhaps completely foreign territory. It may make you feel a little uncomfortable or anxious initially because it is totally outside your comfort zone. If that is the case for you, remember that you are basically just trying to clear your mind by doing the physical act of breathing to help you to switch out of that fight or flight part of your nervous system. Eventually you will get to a place where you will not even be consciously thinking about this. You will find yourself automatically doing this over time. It is a great technique.

Do not worry about whether you are successful in achieving a deep level of relaxation. Maintain a passive attitude and permit relaxation to occur at its own pace. When distracting thoughts occur, try to ignore them by not dwelling upon them and return to repeating "one." With practice, the response should come with little effort. Practice the technique once or twice daily but not within two hours after any meal, since the digestive processes seem to interfere with the elicitation of the *Relaxation Response*. Listen to any soothing, mellifluous sound, preferably with no meaning or association, to avoid stimulation of unnecessary thoughts.

The Mind Body Connection

We have options to put a positive or negative spin on most potentially stressful situations we encounter. We create our own stories.

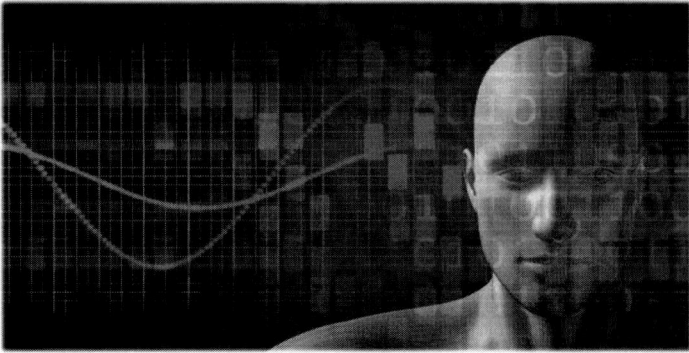

Napoleon Hill, an American presidential advisor and author of the bestselling book *Think and Grow Rich* (1939), wrote about ways to achieve personal success through positive beliefs. Many of his expressions are frequently quoted classics. He stated that "your mental attitude is something you can control outright and you must use self-discipline to create a positive mental attitude" and that "your mental attitude attracts to you everything that makes you what you are" (http://www.azquotes.com/quote/613297).

What are the things that cause you to become stressed? Make a list of things that cause you to stress. What is on the list? Is it your financial situation, your boss, your spouse, your kids, the taxes, the economy, your work commute, traffic or the political situation? Write down everything that causes you to stress out. Do not take any short cuts. Now go through your list and think about things that allow you to put a more positive spin on them. Once you have done that, take each stressor and put a positive spin to it.

For example, suppose you are in traffic and someone cuts you off, you can think that that was not very nice, but then you can rationalize the negative "cutting off" by thinking maybe she was in a rush to get to the hospital because of an emergency or maybe she was having some other issues. Perhaps you are in a hurry and you end up picking the grocery line that ends up moving the slowest because someone at the till is counting a stack of coins or socializing with the cashier. Instead of becoming frustrated and thinking, *"enough already, I'm in a hurry, let's get this thing going,"* think another few minutes is not going to make any difference in my life, so simply look around, notice things around you and relax in the situation. So, in terms of stress, much comes down to choice. It is always your choice.

There is always something that leads someone to do something that results in a stressful situation. It is your choice, however, to deal with it in a way that creates the least amount of stress for you. You can choose to deal with those issues by putting a more positive spin on them, rather than by getting angry or frustrated and consequently further increasing your stress level. We get to choose whatever story we want to place around an event. So, you can create all kind of stories from that outcome or event. That's your choice.

To Think Is To Create

It is not the event that stresses you out, rather it is how you choose to think about that event.

It is not the event that stresses you out, rather it is how you think about the event that stresses you out. How you think creates your experience. You create your own experience around the event. Most people are victims to events and feel like things are happening to them. Is bad traffic the cause of your stress or just traffic?

It is not any of these things that stress you out. It is not the event that stresses you. It is how you think about the event. As Napoleon Hill noted, how you think creates your experience. We have a choice in life to create our own experiences. Although it may be hard for some of you to grasp that thought or that concept. If your thinking is creating your experience, then you can take any event and make anything you want out of it. Most people end up being victims to these events and they feel like things are happening to them, but when you think about it things do not happen to you, rather things just happen and maybe you happen to be there and maybe you participate and maybe you do not.

It is the same thing with other people. You may think that a particular person stresses you out, however, that person is just doing their thing and you get to choose to pay attention or not. It is up to you whether to become victim to their activity or comments. Once you start to realize that in your life you have power over your life, you have power over your level of stress, then you will be able to more easily make choices whether to be stressed out or not. It takes training to change negative patterns. There may be work colleagues or family members that absolutely drive you nuts, but with some work there are things you can do to unlock those stress patterns.

Techniques to Change Stress Patterns

The subconscious mind does not know right or wrong, good or bad.

There are a number of techniques to change our stress patterns and even our belief systems. It is like a muscle memory, like a good golf swing. Some of these stress patterns are deep rooted or illogical. Often we are planting things in our subconscious mind that we are not even aware of and the problem is that our subconscious mind directs our conscious mind in the decisions we make. However, with a bit of work you can learn to break that. It is possible to change new inputs into the conscious mind.

The analogy of the little snowman is a simple way thinking about how the mind works. The conscious mind is you going about your day making conscious decisions and choices. The subconscious often it works in the form of visuals, of pictures. It does not know right or wrong, good or bad. It just says okay to whatever you plant in it.

We put a vast amount of information into our subconscious and over time it creates our belief systems and our stories and at the next level what we might call our infinite, god or spirit or whatever.

The notion that the subconscious mind just says okay to whatever we plant in there is a bit scary and exciting at the same time. It is important to realize that you can plant new programs and belief systems into your subconscious mind and that the subconscious mind during the course of the day is going to influence your decisions.

Visualization Technique

Using mental visualization on a daily basis can help to reduce stress in the body.

Start top of the body, scalp all the way down to toes. If you notice fatigue or tension, visualize it melting away. Work slowly each region as you notice the stress leaving.

There is an accompanying visualization technique audio program that you can download as an MP3. The technique is relatively simple. Close your eyes, then visualize your body relaxing through different stages from the head to the toes. We will get into a bit more depth on that. Once you've listened to it once or twice, you should be able to do it yourself. Visualize as you listen to the audio for the entire ten minutes. Relax and resist the temptation to fast forward.

Being With Technique

Download the accompanying *Being With* Technique audio. Doing this once a day for twenty minutes will equal three hours of sleep in its ability to rejuvenate and to relax you. Try doing this daily for one week and you will be amazed as to how refreshed and rejuvenated and less stressed you feel. You can also try using this technique for five to ten minutes before normally stressful situation like going for a job interview, doing a presentation or even going to the dentist. Also try doing this technique routinely for five minutes before you go to work or immediately upon arriving home. You may find that you will have a much better interaction with your family. Other times when it would be helpful to use this technique would be right before you go to sleep, to generate an energy pick during the day or when you need a creative inspiration.

In Native American culture, they talked about this technique as levelling the water. When a warrior was out in battle or killed an animal, before they could come back into the village they had to stay outside the boundaries of the village, sit down, relax and do some deep breathing to match the water level in the camp. In order for the warriors not to be agitated, they had to calm the water and bring it to the same level. It is a very ancient idea with a lot of current application.

Deep breathing is great because it creates a physiological change in your body immediately. This is going to change how your subconscious mind works. It is going to affect physiology as well. Making this technique a habit will generate more energy as well. Maybe every afternoon instead of heading for the coffee maker because you are feeling fatigued, try this instead. It will not put you to sleep, rather it will likely give you an energy boost and trigger some creativity. If you are stumped on a business project or on the final chapter of a book you are trying to finish writing, this technique will help your subconscious mind go into a state of relaxation to assist the creative juices to flow.

Tapping Technique to Combat Stress and Anxiety

There are a number of different names that have been used for this technique, but they are basically very similar. This technique has been referred to as the emotional freedom technique, the meridian tapping technique or the thought field therapy technique. Basically this technique entails tapping on acupuncture meridian points when you are thinking of certain thoughts. It has often been used to alleviate pain or phobias that may affect your stress levels and underlying health. A phobia of water, of flying, of heights, or of speaking in public are just some of the areas that this technique may help to alleviate. The video will walk you through the tapping technique steps. This technique is another way to break through some of those hard-wired emotions. For those neurological patterns that have developed in your body, it is an effective way to break through those negative patterns.

You can also refer to the links, www.emofree.com, www.rogercalahan.com for additional information.

The Inner Ring; Outer Ring Concept

There may be those situations where you simply cannot find a single technique to help you to deal with a person in your life who has been a source of on-going stress for you. You just cannot figure out right now how to deal with the person. Perhaps in time you will figure it out, but for the time being you need some space. This is when we recommend you try using the inner ring outer ring concept.

Perhaps the source of this stress is an old drinking buddy, a work colleague or an ex-spouse. There is something about them that always bring you down. Every time you are around them you feel like you have been set back fifteen steps. In these situations, we recommend that you take that individual and think about a target on that inner ring. Think about moving them out a ring or two in your life.

If it is a work colleague or your boss, it may be difficult. However, it is possible to move these people from the inner circle by simply keeping the situation at a purely professional level. Reserve the inner circle for your close friends and family, for the good people who genuinely care about you, who are there to support you, who are your back up, who help you to get back on track when you are trying to improve your life.

You tend to be as successful as your closest friends and acquaintances. Your pocket book will reflect that as well. Some of the best leaders in the world in history have made a point of having good people around them. That is not to say that you cannot have acquaintances and friends with other people, but reserve the inner circle for the people who really care. Avoid being surrounded by people who stress you out all the time until you can get these techniques down and you feel confident that you can combat that stress.

Download the relaxation response and the pre-recorded component of the *Being With Technique* from http://thewellness solution.co/wp-content/uploads/2013/10/BeingwithTechnique. mp3. We encourage you to do these techniques for seven days, twenty minutes per day and journal or log some of the changes you notice. Have your energy levels improved? Are you sleeping better at night? Are your relationships less edgy or anxious? Make a note of those things. The more you do these techniques, the more successful you will become in breaking through some of these deep-rooted emotional patterns. You will find that you are going to get through these situations much easier. Some of the great masters of our time, have utilized versions of these techniques.

The longer you do these exercises, the more beneficial the results. John Kehoe's analogy of a well pump presents a good analogy (http://www.learnmindpower.com/). When you first start pumping for water, you may not get any water. It may take a number of pumping actions before the water starts to flow out. Once it starts flowing, it will continue to flow as long as you continue to pump. However, if you stop the process for any length of time, you are going to have to start that process all over again. Similarly, if you get into the habit of doing these techniques on a regular basis you will get on-going, improved results.

Often in our lives we like to treat symptoms and when the symptoms get better we stop doing the things that resulted in the improvements. Once you get to a place where you have alleviated your stress, do not stop doing the techniques or you may end up where you started from. It is all about consistency, whether, it is diet or exercise, or stress management. It is all about that consistency.

Chapter 11

The Nervous System and Wellness: Understanding How They Relate Will Lead to Optimal Health

Our bodies interface with the world through our nervous system.

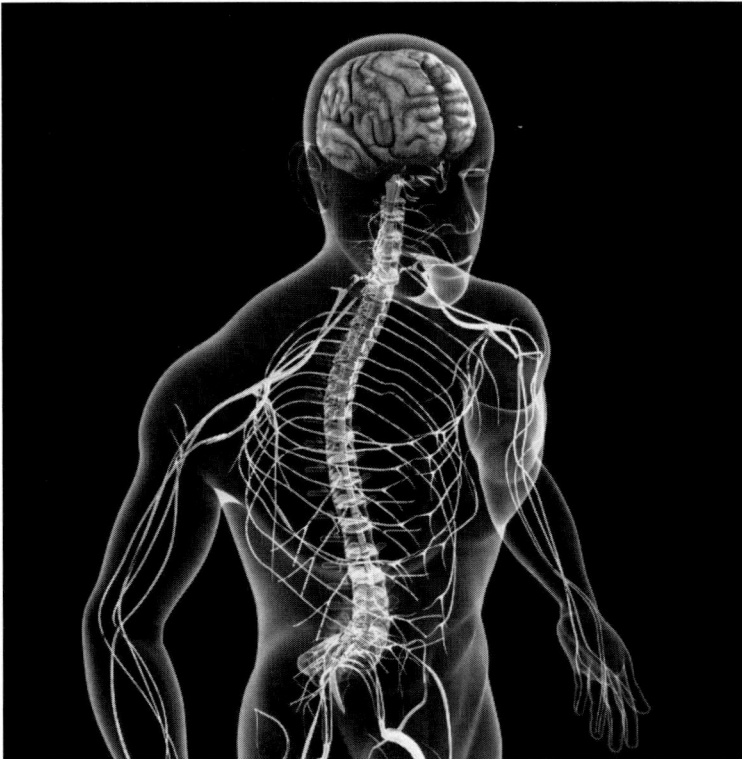

In this eleventh chapter, we explore in a simple and easy to understand way, how this master control system known as our nervous system works. Our bodies interface with the world through our nervous system. All incoming stimulus and environmental change is received and filtered through this nervous system. Our nervous system then produces the appropriate adaptation and change in our bodies. This beautiful exchange of information between the brain and body and body and brain is what keeps us alive, adaptable to the environment and healthy. Any breakdown in this communication can be devastating to our health.

The Nervous System

All incoming stimulation from the outside world is received through our nervous system.

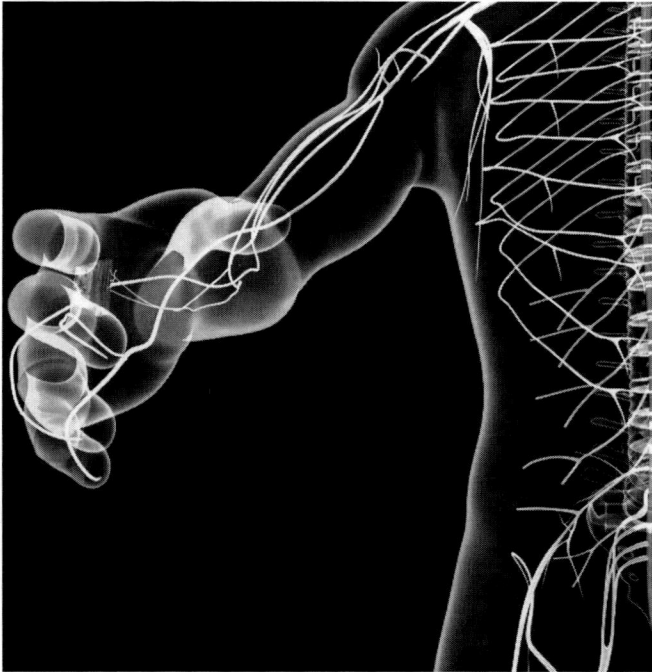

When we talk about our nervous system, what specifically are we talking about? What is our nervous system? Here is a simple definition: *"the bodily system that in vertebrates is made up of the brain and spinal cord, nerves, ganglia, and parts of the receptor*

*organs and **that receives and interprets stimuli and transmits impulses to the effector organs**.*" (http://www. merriam-webster.com/dictionary/nervous%20system)

Our nervous system is basically how our bodies interface with the world around us. We are our nervous system. If we did not have our nervous system, we would be a big glob of cells with no way to know what is happening in our environment and that is obviously a pretty big deal.

All incoming stimulus and environmental change is received and filtered through our nervous system. Light, sound, taste, all types of touch sensation (vibration, pressure, hot, cold, dull, soft, pain, body position awareness, internal body changes in the gut, lungs, heart, hormones, etc. So, when we look at the job of the nervous system and think about our adaptability to our environment, it basically all comes down to all that incoming stimulation from the outside world. This stimulation comes in and is received through our nervous system through all the different nerve receptors in our skin, in our eyes, in our joints, in our muscles, even on our organs, so all that sensory stimulation from the outside world, wind blowing, a certain smell, a cat meowing, stepping on a thumb tack, all those different sensations are running through the nervous system and interpreted through the nervous system, so it is that input and that integration that allows us to adapt to our environment.

Our nervous system then produces the appropriate adaptation and changes in our bodies. Pupils constrict or dilate, heart beats faster or slower, muscles contract or relax, pancreas releases insulin, blood vessels constrict or dilate, our body shivers or sweats.

In every situation your nervous system makes it possible for you to adapt to the environment.

So, talking about adaptation, why is that such a big deal, why do we need to adapt to our environment? What would happen if we didn't adapt to our environment? Well, let us assume that you went outside and it was five degrees Fahrenheit and that your body could not adapt by shivering. The consequence would be that you probably would not last very long. It is the nervous system that makes it possible for your body to adapt to that cold stimulus to warm up your body. A similar process takes place when you go to a hot environment. Your body adapts to cool yourself down.

So, in every situation related to our environment, you are going to have to have that adaptation response for your body to be able to function optimally. It is the job of the nervous system to control that. Most of us have a nervous system that is functioning fairly well, so we do not think about or are not aware of the mechanics of what is taking place in order for our body to adapt to differing environmental conditions.

A great example is Christopher Reeves, the American actor who played the comic book hero, Superman during the 1970s and 1980s. As a result, of a horse riding accident, he had a brain stem injury. He fractured the very top part of his neck and that damaged the spinal cord cutting off much of the communication between the brain and the body, particularly the autonomic nervous system. This resulted in his body no longer being able to adapt to certain situations, temperature being one of them. I remember reading a story where he could not even be wheeled out to the back patio into the sun because he could not sweat to cool himself down. Consequently, he had to remain in a climate controlled home because his body could not adapt to the temperature changes in his environment. His central nervous system simply had no clue as to what was happening in the outside world as the communication could not get through. Likewise, if the house was too cold, he was running into the same situation. He would not be able to warm himself up, so he had a lot of ventilators because the nerves that controlled his lungs were not working properly in addition to a host of other problems.

Fortunately, most of us will not encounter an injury like that in our lifetime, but we may encounter different stressors or problems that can cause those interferences in our nervous system so that we end up not being as adaptable as we should be. Most people take the nervous system for granted because they do not see it and do not realize what is going on so they do not realize when something is not working. We are often unaware when there may be some sort of interference to the nervous system where the stressors to the body have overwhelmed the body's ability to adapt.

Some other examples of appropriate adaptation would be when you walk into a dark room and your pupils dilate or when you go outside on a sunny day and your pupils constrict. Your heart beats faster if you are jogging or running, your skeletal muscles may contract or relax when picking something up, your pancreas may release insulin in the event your blood sugar is higher than it should be, blood vessels may constrict if you are shivering to create heat and expand if you are too hot. The interaction of our body and nervous system is truly a marvelous exchange.

The exchange of information between the brain and the body and the body and the brain is what keeps us alive and healthy.

The beautiful exchange of information between the brain and the body and the body and the brain is what keeps us alive, adaptable to the environment and healthy. Any breakdown in this communication can be devastating to our health. The breakdown in communication between the brain and the body is called nerve interference. We like to think of this as a very beautiful exchange between the information in the outside world getting to the brain through the body and then the brain then processing that information. Then the central nervous system creates an output to the body to say that this is what I need you to do.

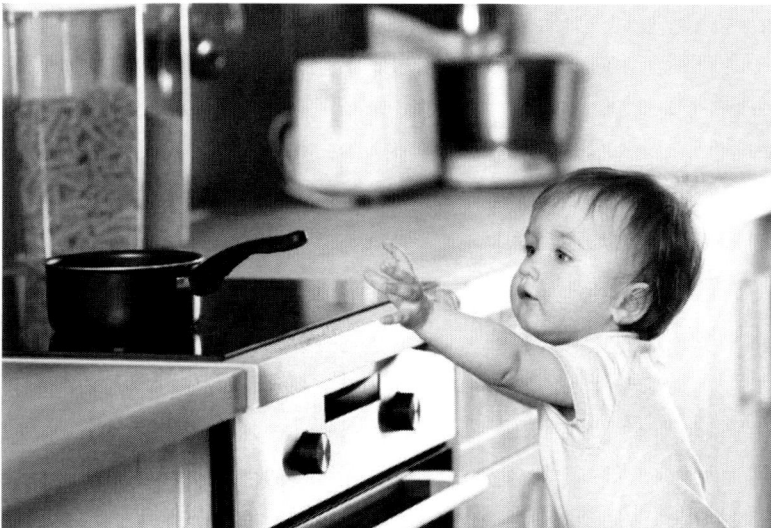

For instance, assume that you touch a hot plate or a hot element on the stove, the sensors in your fingers detect that your fingers have touched something hot and send a message to the brain. The brain then declares the surface your fingers have touched is hot and likely to burn your fingers. This triggers a reflex in the spinal cord resulting you pulling your hand away by contracting your bicep muscle. Amazingly, all this happens in milliseconds. It is incredible how this process happens all day long, every moment of the day and we do not even think about it.

203

Any breakdown in that communication between the brain and the body can be devastating to our health, not necessarily that second, but eventually. It can happen even with minor interference. Pressure on a nerve is enough to cause interference and the longer the pressure remains on the nerve, the worse interference gets. Eventually, the nerve can start to atrophy and scar tissue can form. Often we may not notice that initially, but often it may show up initially as a little bit of numbness or tingling, or it could be some kind of chronic intestinal problem because the intestines are controlled by the nerves. Instead, more likely, we blame the issue it on some sort of a disease rather than an interference in the communication by the nervous system.

Every part of the body is controlled by the nervous system, so just little things over time that you may not even notice could start to deteriorate until one day you realize that you cannot even walk up the stairs properly without huffing and puffing because of this built-up nerve interference rather than because of a lung problem.

Three Nerve Analogy: Sensory, Motor, Autonomic

Your nerves reach and influence every single cell in your body.

The three-nerve analogy is a simple way to describe how the nervous system works. There are basically three main branches to the nervous system, the sensory branch the motor branch and the autonomic branch. This is just over simplified neurology 101, if you will. Those three nerves all start in the brain, transmit down as nerve tracks through the spinal cord and then somewhere along the line, they branch out and turn through the peripheral nerves to every cell of the body. So, if you were to take any nerve of the body, splice it open, it would look like a fiber optic cable with hundreds, if not thousands of fibers in that nerve transmitting information both ways.

Sensory Nerves

The sensory side is what most of us think of when we think about the nervous system. It is taste, touch and smell with again all the information from the outside going to the brain. It is a one-way track, from the outside in. That is the sensory in a nut shell.

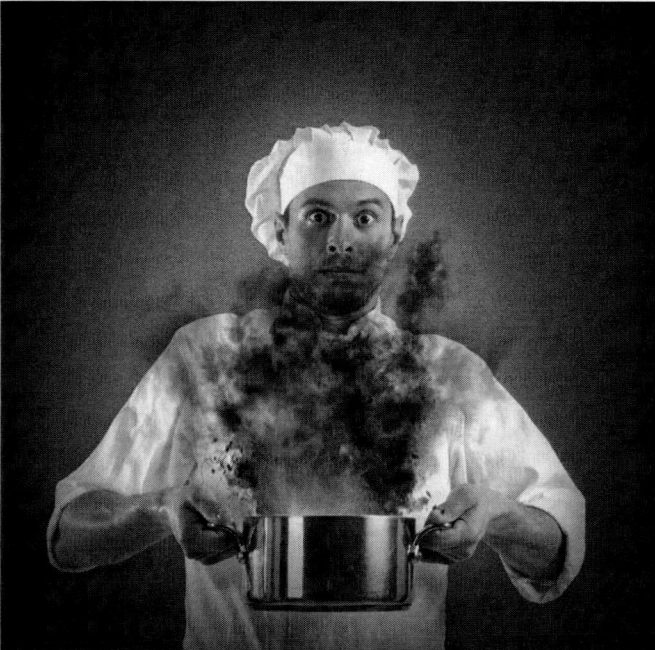

The sensory nerves detect heat of a hot pot

Motor Nerves

Now the motor side, runs from the motor cortex of the brain to the skeletal muscles. It is used to contract the muscles. If you are going to stand up from a chair, lift some weights, move any part of your body, then those are the motor nerves causing the muscles to contract. So again, it is a one-way track from the brain to the muscle.

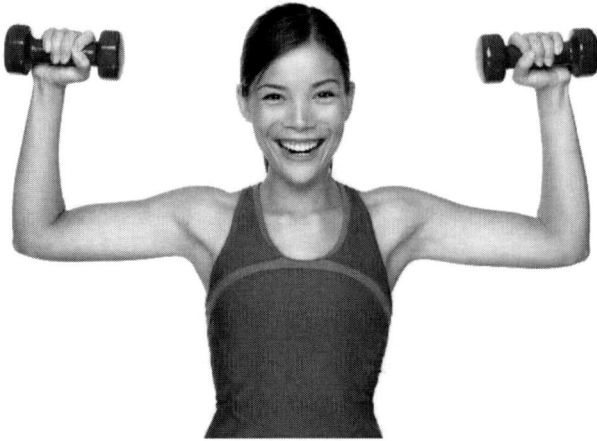

Motor nerves cause muscles to contract

Autonomic Nerves

With the autonomic nervous system, it is the automatic regulation of all the bodily functions such as the digestion, heart rate, blood vessels, pupils contracting and dilating, the pancreas releasing insulin, sweat production, and so on. It is all automatic. You do not have to think about it, but it has to happen for you to adapt to your environment.

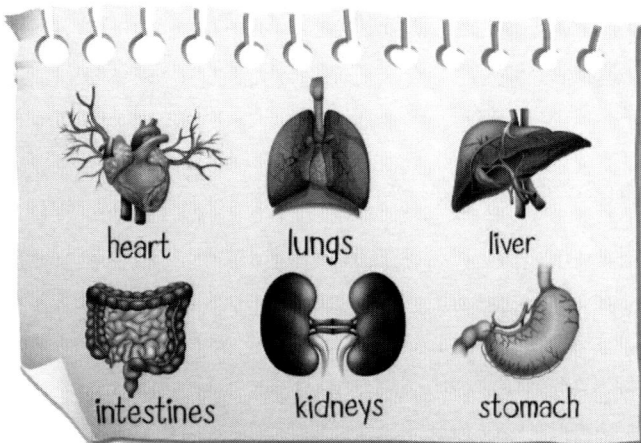

Autonomic nerves control all the organs, glands and blood vessels

Imagine if you had interference on one of those nerves, let us say it is the sensory nerve and ended up with only fifty per cent of the nerve flow coming through, what would happen? For purposes of this illustration, let us say it is the nerve that controls the skin of your hand. You may then end up having some tingling or numbness in your hand around that interference. Or if the nerve damage is severe, you may end up having numbness so you cannot feel the area at all. The sensation would be similar to the dentist giving you a shot that results in complete lack of feeling and communication blockage to the nerve. Although this would not be life threatening, it would alter the quality of your life. Diabetics can have the same sensation when they end up with neuropathy or nerve damage to one or both feet. Obviously, this can be a serious problem.

The second nerve, the motor nerve transports information to the muscles and is responsible for movements such as contractions and twitching. Imagine if you had a fifty per cent reduction to the nerve that goes to your hand and produces your grip. You may start to notice that you drop your credit card while trying to swipe or tap it at the gas station or you drop your keys or cannot hold on to your coffee cup securely anymore, well that could be a reduction of communication to that nerve.

Suppose you have an irritation to the nerve resulting in too many signals to the brain. This could create hyper excitement with muscles going into uncontrollable spasms. So, it is not the muscle that has gone bad, rather it is the nerve telling the muscle that it is not working properly. Then like in Christopher Reeves' spinal cord injury scenario, the skeletal muscles start to atrophy and waste away. There is no longer any control of those muscles, nor any movement at all. Christopher Reeves did not have a muscle injury, rather he had a nerve injury. The muscles were just doing what they are told. If they cannot get the information, they simply waste away.

The autonomic nerves go to all the organs, glands and blood vessels. Let's give an example of the nerve that goes to your stomach. What happens if you irritate this nerve and consequently decrease the flow to that nerve by fifty per cent? What would that look like for your stomach? Perhaps you will end up with chronic indigestion.

On the other hand, if you have too much communication going through that nerve, you may experience irritability coming through that nerve that could result in chronic acid reflux or heart burn. We have had patients in their twenties who have told us that they have experience heart burn by simply drinking a glass of water and that the acid reflux is so bad they have to sleep on an incline at night. Water does not cause heart burn. There is something unusual about someone in their twenties having acid reflux. There might be some interference going on causing that irritation to the stomach. That could also happen to the nerves going to your heart causing a heart attack, to your lungs causing shortness of breath or asthma, to your pancreas causing diabetes or your gallbladder preventing proper bile excretion.

We could just go on and on looking at these things, so it is important to understand our nervous system controls everything through this system and will not function properly if there is interference. You may not initially feel anything, but it will show up as a health problem sooner or later. A lot of people do not make that connection. They tend to think of the nervous system as the sensory information or the pain information only. If there is a pain, something is wrong, but if it is an organ not functioning properly, or some other part the autonomic nervous system or even muscle tension if it is too tight, they do not make the connection of what is causing it. People just think it is some sort of disease condition that is creating the problem. They do not realize it could be just some nerve interference preventing those organs from working properly.

We ask all our patients what they consider good health to be. Most common response is, "If I feel good then I am healthy". So, a lot of people base their health on whether they have symptoms. If they do not have symptoms, they think they are perfectly healthy, so we always like to ask them what percent of our nervous system are sensory nerves or the ones that you feel with. Perhaps 10 per cent or less depending on what studies or books you look at. So, you could have a problem with ninety per cent of your nervous system but you could not be aware of any particular symptoms that something is going on. It is down the road when you cannot digest your food properly or having asthma symptoms or things like that when you finally start to realize something is going on but there is not this quick response. And it is not normally thought of as being associated with a nerve problem.

Asthma could be a nerve problem and that is why we so many of these chronic conditions not being addressed appropriately and instead you see a lot of unnecessary medications being prescribed and surgeries being performed. These interventions may suppress symptoms, but it will not necessarily cure the underlying problems because those have not been addressed. It is the underlying issues, the stressors and things that cause those conditions that must be addressed.

Causes of Nerve Interference

If health is defined as functioning at 100%, then we must also have fully functioning communication between the brain and the body with zero interference.

Physical injury, such as whiplash, nerve compression or concussion, biochemical issues from medications, toxins in food, preservatives or poor hydration and emotional stress, such as anger, resentment or hate can all cause nerve interference. If health is defined as functioning at 100%, then we must also have fully functioning communication between the brain and the body with zero interference.

So, what causes nerve interference? Well it could be any type of physical, biochemical or emotional stress your body is unable to handle. It is important to point out that it does not have to be the physical injury as most people assume, rather it can be any of these stressors. If you have been in a car accident and you have had a brain injury, then that obviously results in nerve interference. If you have had whiplash in the neck causing irritation on the nerves, you will likely experience numbness and tingling, maybe weakness in your hands or spasms in your shoulders. Additionally, the daily medication you take can cause multiple side effects. Some medications cause creates irritation on the nerves or interference of the nervous system resulting in communication breaking down.

As mentioned, previously mentioned, toxins and preservatives in our foods or not being properly dehydrated can cause nerve interference. The nervous system is carefully balanced with certain levels of hydration, certain types of healthy fats and if those go out of sync, even slightly in certain cases that then can cause nerve interference. This biochemical imbalance can result in symptoms such as migraines, headaches, numbness and tingling. Emotional stress can be a toxin to the nervous system. We discussed this in our previous chapter. Therefore, it is very important to learn how to deal effectively with negative emotional triggers. If you are in a toxic environment emotionally, that is toxic to the nervous system and eventually it will take its toll.

Home Nerve System Checks

To be truly healthy you need to have fully functioning communication between the brain and the body which means zero interference of the nerves or nervous system. So how can we determine where we are at? There are some simple home nerve system checks you can do on your own that we have used in our practice. Three of these are, the partner assisted side evaluation posture check, the front posture evaluation and the bilateral weight scales. Except for two weight scales and a camera, you do not need any equipment or technology.

The partner assisted side evaluation posture check

Normal	Your Posture from Side

Your Posture Viewed from the Side

Your head weighs approximately 9.8 lb and is shifted 0.60" forward

Based on physics, your head now effectively weighs 15.6 lb instead of 9.8 lb

Shoulders are shifted 0.57" backward

Hips are not shifted significantly

Knees are not shifted significantly

PAIN SCALE

0 1 2 3 4 5 6 7 8 9 10

During this assessment, you noted that your pain was 0 out of 10 (worst possible pain). Remember that pain and symptoms can be directly associated with abnormal faulty body structure - ie. Abnormal Posture

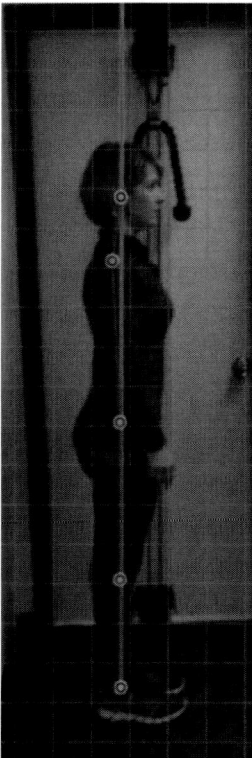

This is a simple check that can be performed simply by someone standing next to you. Look straight forward standing in a posture that is comfortable for you. Have a partner look at you from the side and then have the person draw an imaginary line from your ear straight down to the ground. It should fall through to the middle of your shoulder, middle of your hip, middle of your knee, down through the large bump on the side of your foot. If it does not fall through all those points, there is some interference that is causing an imbalance. Unless this is addressed, depending how progressive it is, it could cause some permanent changes. This is a simple check to see if you have something going on, but obviously if it appears that there is an issue, you need to see a professional.

The front posture evaluation

Your Posture Viewed from the Front
Head is not shifted significantly left or right and is tilted 4.5° left
Shoulders are not shifted significantly left or right and are not tilted
Ribcage is shifted 0.50" right
Hips are not shifted significantly left or right and are tilted 2.6° left

Any measurable deviation from normal posture causes weakening of the spine as well as increased stress on the nervous system which can adversely affect overall health.

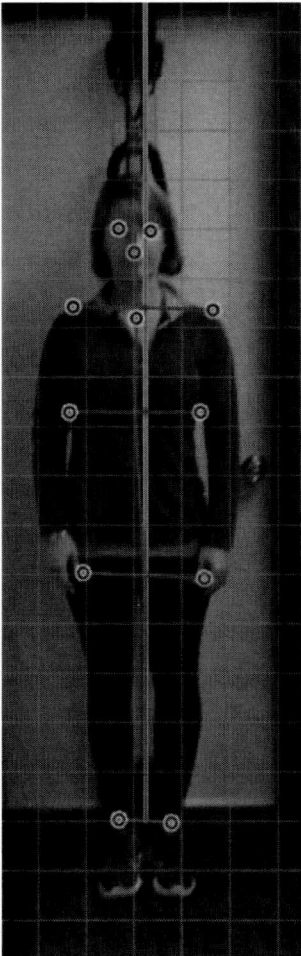

There are several relatively inexpensive posture evaluation apps you can download to your phone, IPad or computer. Simply do a google search to explore the options. You do not need an app to do this however. The posture evaluations generally look for distortion, such as the head is tilting to one side indicating imbalance in muscle tone, symmetry or interference in the nervous system. Although this does not take the place of a professional analysis, it might be a fun thing to do. You might want to try it out on your kids or your spouse, but again it is not a conclusive diagnostic test for what is going on. It is simply a quick way to do a check. Alternatively, you can just take a front digital photo of yourself, then with a sharpie, place a dot on the top of each shoulder, the top of each knee, the outside of each ankle and the nose sternum. Then draw a line to connect the dots. So, what you are looking for are distortion, maybe the head is tilting to one side, again indicating imbalance in muscle tone, symmetry, interference in the nervous system

The Bilateral Weight Scales

The bilateral weight scales can produce a lot of good information. Place two identical scales on the floor approximately six inches apart. Place one foot on each of the scales. Look straight ahead, take a few breaths in and out while standing balanced and comfortable. Then look down and get a reading. It may be easier to have someone look at the dials on the scale for you. Are you heavier on one scale over the other than the other? How you carry yourself and how you distribute your weight can be representative of imbalance in the nervous system. If your weight is not evenly distributed over your feet, you are going to have problems walking and doing various tasks requiring mobility

Checking the nervous system well before symptoms appear is important especially in children to prevent problems from progressing into chronic health issues. Children may or may not complain about nerve or health problems if they are asymptomatic. Whether they do or do not, they can have interference from childbirth, such as trauma to the head or neck, that can progress and as they grow may lead to chronic ear infections and hearing problems as an example. It is always wise to look at preventive approaches to prevent the problem from developing in the first place.

For comprehensive analyses of nerve function interference, it is best to seek out a professional practitioner. If you are wanting to get a much more sensitive nervous system function test, we recommend you seek out a practitioner who uses the Insight Subluxation Station. You can do a google search for chiropractors in your area and ask if they scan your nervous system to look for interference. What you would be looking for would be parameters that measure different nervous system functions such as muscle tone and tension, thermal test that looks at autonomic nervous system function through temperature variations and the pain and sensitivity part of the nervous system. You may also want to look for someone that has a pulse wave profiler that measures heart rate variability to look for balance in autonomic nervous system function to the heart. These tests are a way to take a fairly complex nervous system and measure certain parameters to see if there is interference and then decide where the interference is coming from and whether it is something that can be addressed.

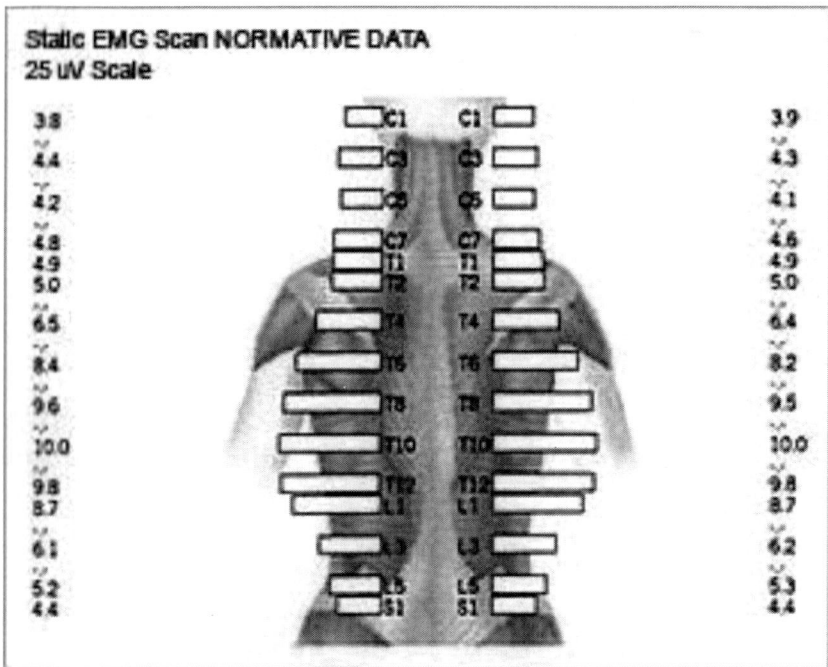

Static EMG Scan NORMATIVE DATA
25 uV Scale

Normal Function
White Bars

Sample Motor Nerve Scan Using Insight Subluxation Station, Showing Normal Function

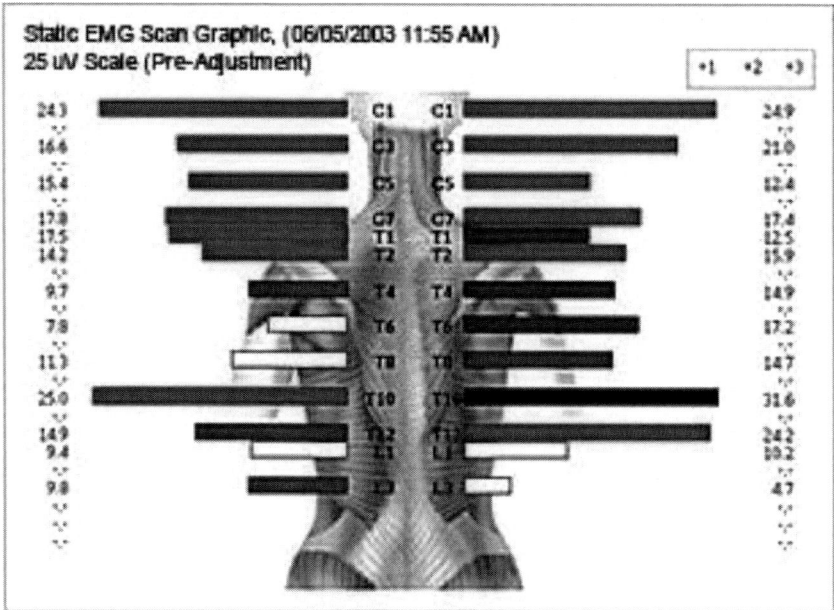

Static EMG Scan Graphic, (06/05/2003 11:55 AM)
25 uV Scale (Pre-Adjustment)

Abnormal Function

Mild/Green Bars
Moderate/Blue Bars
Severe/Red Bars

Sample Motor Nerve Scan Using Insight Subluxation Station, Showing Abnormal Function

In this chapter, we looked at the nervous system, how amazingly it works and some of the consequences when interference between the brain and the body's communication system breaks down. We suggest that you consider doing a self-evaluation, and if you think it is appropriate for you, see a practitioner who specializes in this area for a more detailed analysis. Think about those areas in your life that could be causing interference, poor posture, poor diet, lack of exercise, lack of stretching, medications you are taking. Assess your options and make appropriate changes. By now you may have made some changes, but after reading this you may choose to address some other areas to work on as well. Prevention is always going to be better than treating a problem, so stop it before it happens. Again, we do not live in a bubble. Health is a continuum so the promises you make today are going to change your health tomorrow and the choices you make tomorrow will change your health the next day so it is a day by day process. Sometimes if you wait too long you can no longer reverse the damage. You are definitely going to want to start sooner than later.

Chapter 12

The Power of Attraction: Simple Steps to Achieve Your Dreams, Wishes and Goals

Purpose gives you the compass to truly change your life for the better.

Purpose is everything. It answers the question of what job you should have, should you get married and to whom, and your involvement in your community and the world. Without purpose, we have no compass or way to navigate life's choices. We tend to jump from one thing to the next or we let other's choices dictate our choices. Without a clear purpose, life just seems to "happen" to us. Discovering your purpose will truly change your life and give you that compass. Once you are clear on your purpose you will be able start attracting your dreams, wishes and goals through the power of attraction.

In this final chapter, we will help you discover YOUR purpose. We will give you effective personal development tools to play the game of life in a much bigger and profound way.

How to Find Your Purpose

Your purpose dictates everything you do in life.

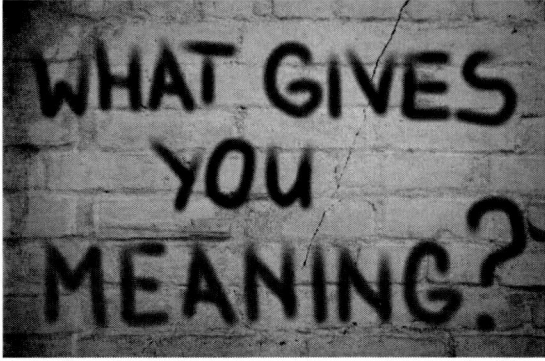

When we are talking about finding your purpose, what is it that we are talking about? It can be a big discussion with many different approaches that can be taken. It is a topic, however, that needs to be taken seriously because your purpose dictates everything you do in life. It is your compass to finding the right path and to maneuvering successfully through the obstacles that may stand in the way to your destination. Your purpose dictates what kind of job you have, what kind of individual you should marry, your involvement in your community and ultimately in the world.

Unfortunately, so many of us, as we go through life, do not have that compass. We do not know what we were put on earth for. A lot of people go through life not knowing what direction they should follow or what they want to accomplish. They just go through the daily routines not knowing what they really want out of life. That is a big reason why people do not get ahead or experience fulfillment in life. When you look at almost every successful person who has achieved what they wanted in life, they have had clarity of purpose. They have known what it is that they have been shooting for and the direction to take to achieve that purpose.

Purpose encompasses a lot of things, including your talents and your interests. It is also connected to your values and beliefs. As you go through life, your purpose can evolve and change. It can become clearer, more precise and perhaps more expansive and ambitious. The material in this chapter is important because it will change you. You will evolve and gain a clarity of purpose that you did not experience before. You will not be the same person you were previously. If you are married or have a partner, it is helpful to try to take share some of this information with them. As you go through your personal development, you may find yourself down the road in a much different place.

Your level of consciousness may be much different, you may be thinking differently than when you first met your partner or spouse, so the more you include your partner in your personal growth plan, the smoother the journey will be. You cannot, of course, force your partner to do something she or he is not comfortable with. Do not bang the Wellness Solution over their head, rather simply share the information and your plans. Have conversations with your partner, as well as your children. If you go to seminars, offer them the option to participate. If you are listening to tapes in the car, there are a lot of things your kids will pick up on. You may not realize that they are listening until they start to ask questions. If you can give them that gift at a young age, by the time they are in high school and college, they could have a clearer sense of who they are as an individual and that can be powerful.

Clarifying Your Purpose: Two Assessment Tests

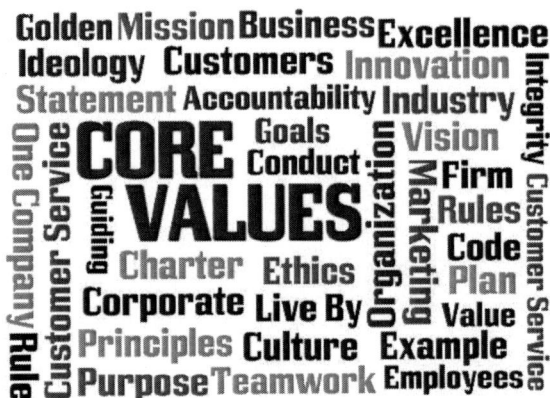

Golden Mission Business Excellence
Ideology Customers Innovation
Statement Accountability Industry
One Company Rule Customer Service Guiding CORE Goals Conduct VALUES Charter Ethics Corporate Live By Principles Culture Purpose Teamwork Organization Marketing Vision Firm Rules Code Plan Value Example Employees Integrity Customer Service

There is a large array of materials you can pursue to help you to clarify your purpose in life. Here are a couple of resources that we have found interesting. The first is the Passion Test by Janet and Chris Atwood and the second is the Personality Style Profile by Anthony Robbins.

The Passion Test

Janet and Chris Atwood's *The Passion Test: The Effortless Path to Discover Your Life Purpose (2008)* was popularized when they were guests on the Oprah show some years back. They have a website with a neat online test called the Passion Test (https://www.amazon.com/Passion-Test-Effortless-Discover ing-Purpose/dp/0452289858/). The intent of this test is to assist you to discover your five key passions to help you to direct your life towards those passions. The primary purpose of the questions from this test is to elicit thought.

Do not spend a whole lot of time thinking about the questions, rather, throw out the first thing that pops into your head. These questions are simply intended to bring out who you are, your core. Do not over think the questions. Write down whatever answers initially come to mind. Then see if there is a connection in your responses. You might notice a trend or pattern towards fitness, a trend towards writing a book, maybe a trend towards being politically active, or whatever and realize that you simply have not done anything with these interests. We obviously recommend you start looking into those things. If you were in a certain situation what would you end up doing? If you are going to read a book, what kind of book would it be? The answers to those questions can often point to who you are as an individual and then ultimately to what your purpose is in life.

For example, if as a child, you dreamed of flying or sailing and you could not pass up a book or movie on the topic, then that may play a role in your life. For myself, when I was younger I really liked fitness and was interested in anything related to that. I participated in sports, exercised a lot and was interested in anything related to wellness and nutrition. So, looking back, I can see those trends as a little trail I have left behind while running towards something. This early interest undoubtedly influenced me to become a wellness practitioner and to share the knowledge I have gained with patients and these books. I enjoy getting up in the morning and reading what is new in the field.

Here are a few examples of questions from the Passion Test to get you started. If you are unsure about your early interests, it may be helpful to ask your parents or someone who knew you as a youth to share their thoughts. We have provided a pdf of this test that you can download.

- When I was a kid I dreamed of...
- I can't pass a book or movie about...
- If I played hooky from work for a week, I'd spend the time...
- Most people don't know this about me.
- If I could start my own how to TV show, it would be about...
- If I were to make a homemade gift, it would be...
- I tried it only once or twice, but I really enjoyed...
- The closest I come to a runner's high is when I'm...
- If I won first prize in the talent show, it would be for...

Personality Style Profile Assessment

(www AnthonyRobbins.com)

Anthony Robbins has created a free on-line personality style self-assessment tool (https://www.tonyrobbins.com/ue/). This is a fifteen-minute on-line test intended to assess your personality type and behavioral style. The main purpose of this test is to assist individuals to increase their self-awareness so that they are better prepared to focus their goals in a way that is compatible with their personality traits and behavioral styles.

We periodically use this disc profile assessment in our line of work as a part of the interview process with prospective employees. Each of the four discs or personality quadrants stands for a different personality style. The test is comprised of a series of questions intended to determine your dominant quadrant or driver personality.

Robbins states that his *Personal Strengths Profile* is based on William Marston's behavioral dimensions (Marston, William M. (1928). *Emotions of Normal People*. K. Paul, Trench, Trubner & Co., https://archive.org/details/emotionsofnormal032195mbp). Over the years, there have been numerous personality theories and assessment tests published. Perhaps among the best known are the theories published by Carl Jung (*Psychological Types, 1923*) and that of Katherine Briggs and her daughter, Elizabeth Briggs Myer who based their theories on the works of Jung. *As with all personality assessments, there are issues related to reliability and validity. None-the-less, they are helpful in providing direction and clarifying your goals.*

Tony Robbins' Personal Strengths DISC Profile

(https://www.tonyrobbins.com/ue/)

To take Tony Robbin's Personal Strengths free online test, go to his website and click on Experiences, then DISC Profile. You will be asked to provide some personal information, such as your name, email address and age. Once you have completed the on-line assessment, you will receive a comprehensive PDF report via email. After you receive your analysis, you may get a follow up email or two, but after that you should not get any future emails from the Robbin's team.

Based on the answers to the questions, your personality traits are then categorized into quadrants. Everyone falls into one of the four DISC personalities: dominant, influencing, steadiness or compliant. The overriding quadrant is going to be your driver personality. The following provides a synopsis of Robbin's personality trait's categories:

Dominant

These are the ones who get things done, but they kind of run over people as they are doing it. They want you to cut to the chase, just give you the cliff notes. They see the person and do not want to hear elaborate stories, rather they just want you to get to the point.

Influencing

Your influencing personality is the expressive life of the party, table dancing type of personality. They are not very organized and tend to leave a wake of chaos behind them. They love people and the more people, the better.

Steadiness

The steadiness personality is an analyzer. This is both of our dominant personality type. We like research articles, numbers, spreadsheets, and so on. We tend to nerd out on that stuff.

Compliant

Most people probably fall into the compliant, amiable personality category. This is an individual who cares about others. They like snuggling and relationships, but in their efforts to please others, they sometimes become overly concerned with what other people think.

Everyone is going to have a combination of these traits, but more dominant towards one and secondary towards another. So, let us look at how some of these combinations translate in this disc profile.

The dominant and influencing personality combinations are the extroverted, optimistic, outspoken types. They are generally more product oriented. They like to see outcomes. What is the thing that we made? The dominant, compliant, on the other hand, are more task oriented. The steadiness, compliant combinations are more introverted and pessimistic. They are more process oriented. They care more about the actual process of doing something and not necessarily the product or outcome at the end. The influencing, steadiness combination are more people oriented. They tend to do better in team in jobs that do not require sticking to the task. They prefer situations that entail interactions with people.

Some personalities will clash a bit. Your compliant personality may clash with a dominant personality. Your influencing, emotional, expressive personality may clash with the steadiness or analytical personality. They do not understand each other and prioritize things differently. One of them has minimal organizational skills and the other lives and dies by organization. Some individuals are going to be hard wired a certain way, while others are a mix. Some individuals might be fairly organized for example, but not to the extent that they nerd out if things are not done just so. They do better with tasks and like to have certain outcomes and things handled in a certain way. So again, knowing that about yourself, can give you more clarity when you are trying to discover what it is you are put on this planet to do.

None of these character traits are bad. We want to make that very clear. It is just how you were born, how you were wired, your upbringing and/or your genetics. It can change over time, but knowing that about yourself and then knowing how you relate to other people can be quite powerful. Trying to estimate what another person is like is a good tool to learn to help you to interact with them in a better way. It may be that some of the most powerful people in history could relate to all four personality styles. For instance, if you are very detail oriented it can be somewhat difficult to relate to someone who is not, but you can to learn how to relate to them and understand them better and that gives you power. So again, when you think of developing your purpose, exercises such as this can help you to develop your self-awareness. After all, you need to know where you are at before you can know where to go and how to get there.

Law of Attraction: How to make it work for you.

People pick up on the non-verbal cues we send out and treat us accordingly.

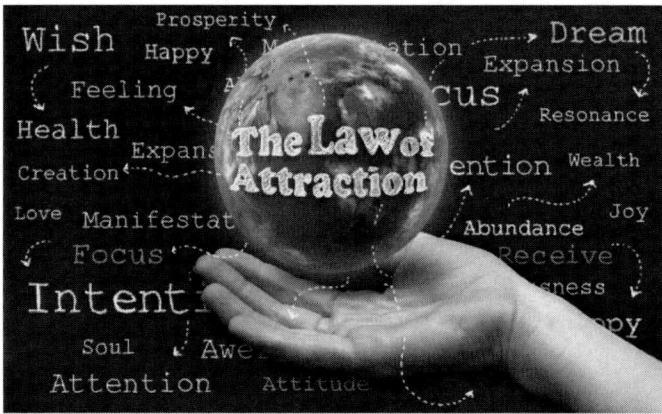

When we talk about finding our purpose in life, the law of attraction fits into that equation. Let us examine the reasoning. The law of attraction basically states that whatever you focus on, you bring into your life. So, what you focus on expands. What you think about now is going to translate into things in your life.

For example, have you ever noticed that when your day starts bad it seems like the whole day goes bad. It is like a self-fulfilling prophecy. Others pick up on our nonverbal cues and projections and treat us accordingly. You have a flat tire when you go out to the car, then you spill coffee on your shirt on your way to work and then you get into an argument with someone at the office. It seems like the whole day kind of snowballs downhill. Sometimes we just chalk that up to a bad day. But the law of attraction would say that because of what you first were thinking about, related to the initial bad situation of the day, you attracted in more of those things throughout the day. For some of us that is kind of an eye opener and for others there may be some skepticism around that.

But there are a lot of situations if you were to look back you might say, "You know what? I can absolutely see that happening. Maybe you can see that happening now. Perhaps you continue to attract the same type of person into your life. You know the people who always seems to attract the alcoholic partners. You wonder what is going on with that situation. Or in a business, it seems every customer who comes in is just difficult to work with, non-compliant, or their checks always bounce. Again, as you focus on that more and more, you may be sending signals out there that can attract that negativity. People are going to start to pick up on that, so that negative or dysfunctional situation will perpetuate or get worse.

Positive people do not want to be surrounded by pessimistic, negative people. Negativity attracts more negativity.

The self-help book and video, *The Secret* ((2006) by Rhonda Byrnes (https://www.amazon.com/Secret-Rhonda-Byrne/dp/) was first popularized on the Oprah Winfrey Show. The book's premise is that through positive thinking you attract positive changes in your life. You attract what you think. Although it is a best-selling book, it has also generated much criticism, mainly that it is pseudo-science and can create false hope.

One thing that was left out of the book was that action was needed as well as positive thoughts. Your positive thoughts may lead to people, places and situations showing up in your life, however, if you don't pick up on this and take action you may miss out on the positive things that were showing up. We are not advocating that you rely solely on positive visualization to achieve your dreams or goals, rather we are saying that by remaining positive you will attract positive, optimistic people around you, view the world as glass half full rather than glass half empty, and that in turn will open doors as you work towards achieving your goals. Let us face it, no one wants to be surrounded by pessimistic, negative people. It is worth watching the video or reading the book regardless of your outlook.

Positive people attract positive people around them.

Non-verbal communication is powerful, just those subtle little clues that you draw around you that you pick up on causing people to act in certain ways around you. Your thoughts are communicated in subtle and sometimes in not so subtle ways by your facial expressions, body language and of course, your speech patterns. So, the key message here is that you need to be mindful of your thoughts because people pick up on that in many different ways.

Mind Power – What Is It? Can You Control It?

Very little in history is completely original. People in each generation

learn, borrow and build on what has transpired in the past.

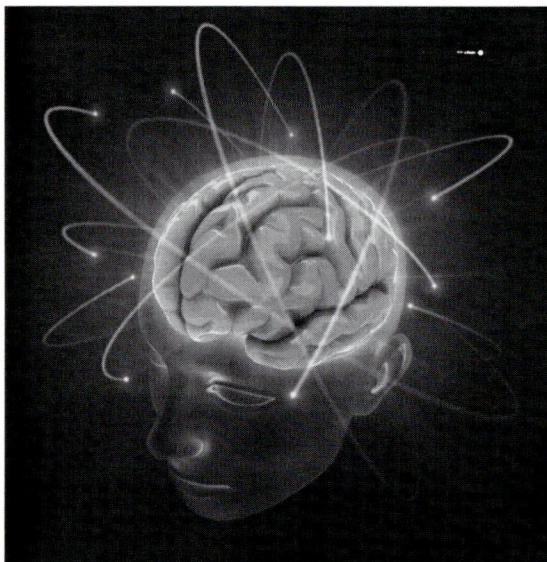

The law of attraction suggests that through the power of positive thinking, you can attract good things into your life. Similar views have been expressed by numerous people and in various formants over the years. Throughout history, influential leaders, philosophers and writers have put forth similar thoughts and inspirational quotes that appear to support wholly or partially the power of positive thinking, which in turn has connections to the law of attraction. Although the views and motivational quotes of these thinkers were not necessarily created specifically with the law of attraction in mind, they none-the-less support the concept of the power of positive thinking and relatedly, its connection to the law of attraction.

Throughout history, influential individuals from various walks of life and backgrounds have spread philosophical similar messages related to the power of positive thinking.

Ideas, in most cases, are not pulled from thin air, rather, ideas are inspired by the writings of the past. Very little in history is completely original. People in each generation learn, borrow and build on what has transpired in the past. It is no different with the current influential theorists who write, lecture and publish motivational quotes related to how the power of positive thinking can help you to achieve the personal and professional growth to attract the positive things to achieve your life goals. Throughout history, influential individuals from various walks of life, religious backgrounds and value systems have spread philosophical similar messages.

Here is a sampling of quotes that span history:

"To find yourself, think for yourself" (circa 470-399 BC Socrates, https://www.goodreads.com/author/quotes/275648. Socrates; www.ancient.eu/socrates/).

"As man thinketh in his heart, so is he". (Proverbs: 23:7, New Testament);

"Be careful how you think. Your life is shaped by your thoughts" (Proverbs: 4:23, New Testament)

"You become what you think about all day long."; "Nothing great was ever achieved without enthusiasm" (1803-1882, Ralph Waldo Emerson, archive.vcu.edu/english/engweb/transcenden talism /authors/emerson/; https://www.goodreads.com/author /quotes/12080.Ralph_Waldo_Emerson)

"If you think you can do a thing or think you cannot do a thing, either way you are right"; "It is not so much whether you can do it or not, it is whether you think you can do it" (1863-1947, Henry Ford, www.biography.com/people/henry-ford) (https://www. brainyquote.com/quotes/authors/h/henry_ford.html;

"People who are unable to motivate themselves must be content with mediocrity, no matter how impressive their other talents". (1835-1919, Andrew Carnegie, www.biography.com/ people/andrew-carnegie; https://www.brainyquote.com/quotes/ authors/a/andrew)

"Positive anything is better than negative nothing" (1856-1915 Elbert Hubbard, www.online-literature.com/elbert-hubbard/; https://www.brainyquote.com/quotes/authors/e/elbert).

"Happiness is when what you think, what you say, and what you do are in harmony" (1869-1948 Mahatma Gandhi, https://www.britannica.com/biography/Mahatma-Gandhi; https://www.brainyquote.com/quotes/authors/m/mahatma)

"A goal without a plan is just a wish" (1900-1944 Antoine de Saint-Exupéry, (https://www.britannica.com/biography/Antoi ne-de-Saint-Exupery; https://www.brainyquote.com/quotes/ authors/a/antoine_de_saintexupery.html)

"You have brains in your head. You have feet in your shoes. You can steer yourself in any direction you choose. You're on your own, and you know what you know. And you are the guy who'll decide where to go". (1904-1991, Dr. Seuss, www.biography.com/people/dr-seuss; https://www.brainyquote .com/quotes/authors/d/dr_seuss.html)

"We become what we think about." "If you think you can do a thing, or think you can't do a thing, your right"; "What the mind of man can conceive and believe, it can achieve" (1883-1970, Napoleon Hill, napoleonhill.wwwhubs.com; https://www.youtube .com/watch?v=oct1UjNetik)

"If you don't know where you are going, you might wind up someplace else" (1925-2015, Yogi Berra, http://www.Spirit button.com/yogi-berra-quotes/).

"Happiness is an inside job"; The pessimist complains about the wind; the optimist expects it to change; the realist adjusts the sails (1921-1994, William Arthur Ward. (https://www. amazon.com/William-Arthur-Ward/; https://www.Brainyquote .com/quotes/authors/w/william_arthur_ward.html).

"Winners learn from the past and enjoy working in the present toward the future"; "There are two primary choices in life: to accept conditions as they exist, or accept the responsibility for changing them". (1933-, Denis Waitley, www.waitley.com/; (https://www.brainyquote.com/quotes/authors/d/denis_waitley. html).

You must believe you can achieve, in order to achieve.

These are all great, basic motivational quotes, but Interestingly the messages in all of them are very similar. How you relate to these messages can have an impact on almost every facet of your life. What they are all saying is that through the power of positive thinking and personal growth, you can attract the supportive people and the requisite things to empower you to achieve your life's goals. Things will change in your life based on what you are thinking and what you believe about those thoughts. Belief is a huge part of what manifests for you. You must believe you can achieve, in order to achieve.

Even if you do not buy into the mythical part of the law of attraction just by focusing on your goals, you are going to do more things to move towards achieving those goals.

We encourage you to start to be more mindful of how your thought process impacts your daily actions and interactions with others. So, what do you do if your thoughts inadvertently turn to the negative? Simply just recognize that that is where your thoughts are going and then redirect those thoughts to what you do want in your life.

Do you wonder about people who just seem to have everything just fall into their lap? Everything seems to go their way. They have been able to accomplish huge things and to make significant contributions. When you look at the backgrounds of these people, you see similar patterns. They believe in themselves, that they can accomplish their goals, their outlook is positive and they have supportive people around them. Of course, you cannot totally dismiss the fact that some of these individuals had the advantage of privileged births and inherited wealth. However, many people have achieved great things without have the kick-start of wealth and powerful connections around them. Additionally, it is unlikely that these individuals who were born into privilege would have been able to accomplish great things without the power of positive thinking and the ability to attract the right people around them to help them to achieve their goals. Through their belief in themselves, they have done the necessary things, advertently and inadvertently, to help them reach their goals.

Law of Attraction Exercise

As we have mentioned, you need to believe you can achieve in order to attract the things in your life to successfully reach your goals. Here is simple exercise that may help you to tweak out your believability around certain things.

Write down ten to fifteen things you would like to see happen in your life or come into your life within the next three to six months. Perhaps you would like to lose twenty pounds, or you want to earn an extra ten thousand dollars, buy a new car, get a new job, or whatever. Next, rate those things from 0-10 as far as whether you believe you can accomplish those things within this time frame. Put a realistic timeline on it. At this point, do not think about how you are going to go about producing these goals, rather just focus on your believability around being able to achieve these goals.

Of course, it is important to keep things realistic. For example, if you currently have only a few thousand dollars and your goal is to obtain $10 million dollars in three months, your believability would likely be low around that. In that case, we recommend you change it or take it off your list. Keep it real because what you believe about that goal is going to predict whether this law of attraction works for you, or not. If you do not believe that you can achieve your goals, your subconscious mind is going to be laughing about it and you will create the opposite effect. You are then going to end up thinking about the lack of having this goal, rather than about having it, which of course is the opposite of what you want to achieve.

Start with little things and then as your believability increases, so will your achievements. Every step you go through is going to increase your believability. It is a snowball effect. Say for instance, you want a new job and as you start thinking about this new job every day, your believability increases. Perhaps you start with a fairly high believability, maybe a seven out of ten. In that case, you are going to go into that process of achieving this goal with some confidence. Once the job materializes, you will begin to feel your believability increasing and with that your confidence in achieving your next goal will also increase. It will be a snowball effect, success building on success.

If you rate something below a five, remove it from your list. Start with the ones six and higher, and then as you achieve your initial goals and your believability goes up, your initial less believable goals will likely be moved up the scale.

As for the actual exercise of thinking about these things, there are a lot of different approaches. I do a lot of this first thing in the morning. I wake up 30 min early and I think about those things I want in my life, focus on each of them for at least 5 minutes or so. I think about how I would feel when it has come into my life and the emotion wrapped up around that. I try to visualize how it would look. Say for instance I want a black jeep, I see the black jeep and I think about how I would feel driving that black jeep. I visualize the surroundings around the jeep, the hills around it, driving through the mountain passes, the jeep in my driveway, or whatever. Again, I try to plant as much as I can into the subconscious mind making the believability that much more powerful.

We recommend a couple of eBooks that you can download. The first eBook, *Think and Grow Rich* (1937) by Napoleon Hill has sold over 100 million copies since it was first published. Hill wrote extensively about personal growth and achievement. His writings and lectures are readily available both in audio and PDF formants on the internet. Hill's influential writings were inspired by the writings of his predecessor, steel magnate and philanthropist, Andrew Carnegie. Carnegie wrote the *The Gospel of Wealth* (1889). He was a self-made millionaire who rose from poverty to become one of the richest people in the world during his lifetime.

The second eBook we have made available for you to download is *The Strangest Secret* by Earl Nightingale (2006). *The Strangest Secret* was an audio record first produced in 1956. His message was greatly influenced by Napoleon Hill's book, *Think and Grow Rich*.

We have also provided you with a link to Martin Boroson's *One-Moment Meditation Technique* (http://www.onemomentmeditation.com). It is a great tool for someone with limited time on their hand to help clear their mind.